Basic Concepts in Pharmacology

Basic Concepts in Pharmacology

What You Need to Know for Each Drug Class

Fourth Edition

Janet L. Stringer, MD, PhD
Dean, Science and Technology
Canada College
Redwood City, California

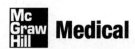
McGraw Hill **Medical**

New York   Chicago   San Francisco   Lisbon   London   Madrid   Mexico City
Milan   New Delhi   San Juan   Seoul   Singapore   Sydney   Toronto

Basic Concepts in Pharmacology: What You Need to Know for Each Drug Class, Fourth Edition

Copyright © 2011 by The McGraw-Hill Companies, Inc. All rights reserved. Printed in the United States of America. Except as permitted under the United States Copyright Act of 1976, no part of this publication may be reproduced or distributed in any form or by any means, or stored in a data base or retrieval system, without the prior written permission of the publisher.

Previous editions copyright © 2006, 2001, 1996 by The McGraw-Hill Companies, Inc.

2 3 4 5 6 7 8 9 0   DOC/DOC   14 13 12

ISBN 978-0-07-174104-0
MHID 0-07-174104-6

This book was set in Times Roman by Glyph International.
The editors were Michael Weitz and Robert Pancotti.
The production supervisor was Sherri Souffrance.
Project management was provided by Ranjit Kaur, Glyph International.
The cover designer was Ashley Lau.
Cover photograph: Drug release in the stomach. (Credit: David Mack/Photo Researchers, Inc.)
RR Donnelley was printer and binder.

This book is printed on acid-free paper.

Library of Congress Cataloging-in-Publication Data

Stringer, Janet L., author.
    Basic concepts in pharmacology : what you need to know for each drug
class/Janet L. Stringer.—Fourth edition.
    p. ; cm.
Includes index.
ISBN 978-0-07-174104-0 (softcover : alkaline paper)
1. Pharmacology—Outlines, syllabi, etc. 2. Drugs—Outlines, syllabi, etc. I. Title.
[DNLM: 1. Pharmacological Phenomena. 2. Pharmaceutical Preparations. QV 4]
RM301.14.S77 2011
615′.1—dc22

                                                                2010043971

McGraw-Hill books are available at special quantity discounts to use as premiums and sales promotions, or for use in corporate training programs. To contact a representative, please e-mail us at bulksales@mcgraw-hill.com.

International Edition ISBN 978-0-07-176728-6; MHID 0-07-176728-2
Copyright © 2011. Exclusive rights by The McGraw-Hill Companies, Inc., for manufacture and export. This book cannot be reexported from the country to which it is consigned by McGraw-Hill. The International Edition is not available in North America.

Key Features of
Basic Concepts in Pharmacology, 4th Edition

A time-saving, stress-reducing approach to learning the essential concepts of pharmacology

- Provides a complete framework for studying—and understanding—the fundamental principles of drug actions
- Simplifies the learning process by presenting drugs by class
- Describes exactly what you must know about each drug class
- Reinforces key concepts and definitions
- Presents important information in convenient boxes, illustrations, and tables
- Points out the concepts you truly must know before moving on to other material
- Helps you organize and condense the drug information you must remember
- Identifies the most important drugs in each drug class
- Great for USMLE review

Presents important drug information in convenient boxes, tables, and illustrations

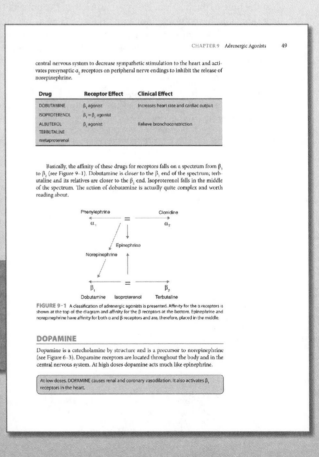

CHAPTER 9 Adrenergic Agonists 49

central nervous system to decrease sympathetic stimulation to the heart and activates presynaptic α_2 receptors on peripheral nerve endings to inhibit the release of norepinephrine.

Drug	Receptor Effect	Clinical Effect
DOBUTAMINE	β_1 agonist	Increases heart rate and cardiac output
ISOPROTERENOL	$\beta_1 = \beta_2$ agonist	
ALBUTEROL	β_2 agonist	Relieve bronchoconstriction
TERBUTALINE		
metaproterenol		

Basically, the affinity of these drugs for receptors falls on a spectrum from β_1 to β_2 (see Figure 9–1). Dobutamine is closer to the β_1 end of the spectrum; terbutaline and its relatives are closer to the β_2 end. Isoproterenol falls in the middle of the spectrum. The action of dobutamine is actually quite complex and worth reading about.

FIGURE 9–1 A classification of adrenergic agonists is presented. Affinity for the α receptors is shown at the top of the diagram and affinity for the β receptors at the bottom. Epinephrine and norepinephrine have affinity for both α and β receptors and are, therefore, placed in the middle.

DOPAMINE

Dopamine is a catecholamine by structure and is a precursor to norepinephrine (see Figure 6–3). Dopamine receptors are located throughout the body and in the central nervous system. At high doses dopamine acts much like epinephrine.

At low doses, DOPAMINE causes renal and coronary vasodilation. It also activates β_1 receptors in the heart.

Adding H⁺ to lower the pH will drive the equilibrium to the right toward the protonated (charged) form. Removing H⁺ to raise the pH will drive the equilibrium to the left toward the uncharged form (unprotonated) of the base (Figure 3–2).

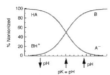

FIGURE 3–2 In this graph the effects of pH on the degree of ionization of both a weak acid and a weak base are presented.

> In the stomach (pH 2.0), weak acids are uncharged and will be absorbed into the bloodstream, whereas weak bases are charged and will remain in the GI tract.

To test your understanding of this, try out these questions. Answers appear at the bottom of the page.*

1. In the intestine (pH 8.0), which will be better absorbed, a weak acid (pK 6.8) or a weak base (pK 7.1)?
2. If we alkalinize the urine to a pH of 7.8, will a lower or higher percentage of a weak acid (pK 7.1) be ionized, compared with when the urine pH was 7.2?

BIOAVAILABILITY

> *Bioavailability* is the amount of drug that is absorbed after administration by route X compared with the amount of drug that is absorbed after intravenous (IV) administration. X is any route of drug administration other than IV.

Example: Suppose you are testing a compound in clinical trials. You have tentatively named this compound "Newdrug." Newdrug is administered orally and plasma levels determine that only 75% of the oral dose reaches the circulation.

*Answers: (1) a weak base; (2) higher, because more weak acid will be ionized the more the pH exceeds the pK.

Reveals effective study techniques not found in any other book

---

40   PART II Drugs That Affect the Autonomic Nervous System

The preceding statement is sweeping and not entirely true. However, the therapeutically useful drugs in reasonable concentrations are muscarinic. The effects of these drugs were listed earlier, but also can be deduced from your knowledge of the parasympathetic nervous system. The differences between the drugs are related to their resistance to cholinesterase activity and specificity for nicotinic receptors.

> BETHANECHOL is used in the treatment of urinary retention.

Of the drugs in this group, bethanechol is the most clinically useful. It is used to treat patients with urinary retention in the postoperative period and in those with a neurogenic bladder.

> The side effects of these drugs are directly related to their interaction with muscarinic receptors.

If you know the actions of these drugs, you also know their side effects. That means there are no new lists to memorize. Side effects often listed for these drugs include sweating (increased secretion), salivation, GI distress, and cramps (due to increased motility).

> Nicotine is a direct agonist at nicotinic receptors.

Nicotine is used therapeutically to help patients stop smoking.

CHOLINESTERASE INHIBITORS

These drugs are often divided into two or three groups based on their structure. Words such as *mono-quaternary amino, bis-quaternary amine, carbamate,* and *organophosphate* appear in many textbooks as names for these subgroups. For our purposes, we'll divide these drugs into two groups: reversible inhibitors, which are water soluble, and irreversible inhibitors (organophosphates), which are lipid soluble.

Reversible Inhibitors		Irreversible Inhibitors
Myasthenia Gravis	**Alzheimer Disease**	
EDROPHONIUM	DONEPEZIL	diisopropyl fluorophosphate
NEOSTIGMINE	galantamine	echothiophate
PYRIDOSTIGMINE	RIVASTIGMINE	isofurophate
ambenonium	tacrine	malathion
demecarium		parathion
physostigmine		sarin
		soman

Identifies the most important drugs in each class

Contents

Preface   xiii

1. WHERE TO START   1

PART **I**

GENERAL PRINCIPLES

2. RECEPTOR THEORY   5
   Agonists   5
   Efficacy and Potency   6
   Therapeutic Index   7
   Antagonists   7
   Inverse Agonists   9

3. ABSORPTION, DISTRIBUTION, AND CLEARANCE   11
   First-Pass Effect   11
   How Drugs Cross Membranes   11
   Bioavailability   13
   Total Body Clearance   14

4. PHARMACOKINETICS   16
   Volume of Distribution   16
   First-Order Kinetics   17
   Zero-Order Kinetics   19
   Steady-State Concentration   20
   Time Needed to Reach Steady State   21
   Loading Dose   22

5. DRUG METABOLISM AND RENAL ELIMINATION   24
   Liver Metabolism   24
   Renal Excretion   25

PART **II**

DRUGS THAT AFFECT THE AUTONOMIC NERVOUS SYSTEM

6. REVIEW OF THE AUTONOMIC NERVOUS SYSTEM   29
   Why Include This Material?   29
   Relevant Anatomy   30
   Synthesis, Storage, Release, and Removal of Transmitters   32
   Receptors   34
   General Rules of Innervation   35
   Presynaptic Receptors   37

7. CHOLINERGIC AGONISTS   38
   Organization of Class   38
   Direct Cholinergic Agonists   39
   Cholinesterase Inhibitors   40

8. CHOLINERGIC ANTAGONISTS   43
   Organization of Class   43
   Muscarinic Antagonists   43
   Ganglionic Blockers   45
   Neuromuscular Blockers   45

9. ADRENERGIC AGONISTS   47
   Organization of Class   47
   Direct-Acting Agonists   48
   Dopamine   49
   Indirect-Acting Agents   50
   Cardiovascular Effects of Norepinephrine, Epinephrine, and Isoproterenol   50

10. ADRENERGIC ANTAGONISTS   52
Organization of Class   52
Central Blockers   52
α-Blockers   52
β-Blockers   54
Mixed α- and β-Blockers   55

PART III
DRUGS THAT AFFECT THE CARDIOVASCULAR SYSTEM

11. ANTIHYPERTENSIVE DRUGS   59
Organization of Class   59
Diuretics   60
Drugs That Interfere With the
  Renin-Angiotensin System   62
  Angiotensin-Converting Enzyme (ACE)
    Inhibitors   62
  Angiotensin II Receptor Blockers (ARBs)   63
  Selective Aldosterone Receptor Antagonists   64
Direct Renin Inhibitor (DRI)   64
Calcium Channel Blockers   64
Nitrates   65
Other Direct Vasodilators   66
α- and β-Blockers   66
Clonidine   67

12. DRUGS USED IN ISCHEMIC HEART
  DISEASE AND CONGESTIVE
  HEART FAILURE   69
Ischemic Heart Disease   69
Congestive Heart Failure   69
Reduction of Cardiac Workload   70
Control of Excessive Fluid   70
Enhancement of Contractility   71
  Cardiac Glycosides   71
  Sympathomimetics   72
  Phosphodiesterase Inhibitors   72
  Ranolazine   72

13. ANTIARRHYTHMIC DRUGS   73
Organization of Class   73
Class I Drugs (Sodium Channel Blockers)   74
Class II Drugs (β-Blockers)   75
Class III Drugs (Potassium Channel Blockers)   76
Class IV Drugs (Calcium Channel Blockers)   77
Other Antiarrhythmic Drugs   78
Drugs That Increase Heart Rate   78

14. DRUGS THAT AFFECT BLOOD   79
Organization of Class   79
Antiplatelet Agents   79
Anticoagulants   81

Thrombolytic Drugs   83
Phosphodiesterase Inhibitors   84
Drugs Used in the Treatment of Anemia   84

15. LIPID-LOWERING DRUGS   86
Organization of Class   86
Additional Explanation of Mechanisms   87

PART IV
DRUGS THAT ACT ON THE CENTRAL NERVOUS SYSTEM

16. DRUGS USED IN DEMENTIA   91
Organization of Class   91
Cholinesterase Inhibitors   91
NMDA Blocker   92

17. ANXIOLYTIC AND HYPNOTIC DRUGS   93
Tolerance and Dependence   93
Organization of Class   94
Barbiturates   95
Benzodiazepines   96
Buspirone   98
Benzodiazepine Receptor Agonists   98
Melatonin Receptor Agonist   98

18. DRUGS USED IN MOOD DISORDERS   100
Organization of Class   100
Serotonin-Specific Reuptake Inhibitors (SSRIs)   101
Serotonin/Norepinephrine Reuptake
  Inhibitors (SNRIs)   102
Heterocyclics/TCAs   102
Monoamine Oxidase (MAO) Inhibitors   103
Other Antidepressants   104
Drugs Used in Bipolar Disorder   105

19. ANTIPSYCHOTICS OR NEUROLEPTICS   106
Organization of Class   106
Typical Antipsychotics (First Generation)   107
Serotonin-Dopamine Antagonists (Second
  Generation)   108
Neuroleptic Malignant Syndrome   109

20. DRUGS USED IN PARKINSON DISEASE   110
Organization of Class   110
Dopamine Replacement Therapy   111
Dopamine Agonist Therapy   112
Anticholinergic Therapy   112

21. ANTIEPILEPTIC DRUGS   113
Organization of Class   113
Important Details About the Most
  Important Drugs   114
Other Drugs to Consider   115

22. NARCOTICS (OPIATES)   117
    Organization of Class   117
    Actions of Morphine and the Other Agonists   118
    Distinguishing Features of Some Agonists   119
    Opioid Antagonists   120
    Opioid Agonist-Antagonists   121

23. GENERAL ANESTHETICS   122
    Organization of Class   122
    Uptake and Distribution of Inhalational
        Anesthetics   123
    Elimination of Inhalational Anesthetics   124
    Potency of General Anesthetics   124
    Specific Gases and Volatile Liquids   124
    Specific Intravenous Agents   125

24. LOCAL ANESTHETICS   126
    Organization of Class   126
    Mechanism of Action   127
    Special Features About Individual Agents   127

PART V
CHEMOTHERAPEUTIC AGENTS

25. INTRODUCTION TO CHEMOTHERAPY   131
    Approach to the Antimicrobials   131
    General Principles of Therapy   131
    Definitions   132
    Important Concepts to Understand   132
    Classification of Antimicrobials   134

26. INHIBITORS OF CELL WALL SYNTHESIS   136
    General Features   136
    β-Lactams   136
        Penicillins   138
        Cephalosporins   139
        Carbapenems   140
        Monobactams (Aztreonam)   140
    Other Inhibitors of Cell Wall Synthesis   141
        Vancomycin   141
        Bacitracin   141
        Fosfomycin   141
        Daptomycin   141

27. PROTEIN SYNTHESIS INHIBITORS   142
    General Features   142
    Aminoglycosides   142
    Tetracyclines   143
    Macrolides   144
    Streptogramins and Oxazolidinones   145
    Chloramphenicol   146
    Clindamycin   146

28. FOLATE ANTAGONISTS   147
    Mechanism of Action   147
    Selected Features   148

29. QUINOLONES AND URINARY TRACT
    ANTISEPTICS   149
    Drugs in This Group   149
    Quinolones   149
    Methenamine   150

30. DRUGS USED IN TUBERCULOSIS AND
    LEPROSY   151
    Organization of Class   151
    Isoniazid   152
    Rifampin   152
    Pyrazinamide   153
    Ethambutol   153
    Dapsone   153

31. ANTIFUNGAL DRUGS   155
    Organization of Class   155
    Azole Antifungals   156
    Polyene Antifungals   157
    Echinocandins   158
    Terbinafine   158

32. ANTHELMINTIC DRUGS   159
    Organization of Class   159
    Drugs Used Against Cestodes and
        Trematodes   159
    Drugs Used Against Nematodes   160
    Drugs Used Against Filaria   160

33. ANTIVIRAL DRUGS   162
    Organization of Class   162
    Anti-HIV Drugs   163
    Drugs Used in Influenza   164
    Other Antivirals   165

34. ANTIPROTOZOAL DRUGS   166
    Organization of Class   166
    Metronidazole   167
    Antimalarial Agents   167
    Therapeutic Considerations   168
    Special Features   168

35. ANTICANCER DRUGS   170
    Organization of Class   170
    Terminology and General Principles
        of Therapy   171
    Adverse Effects   173
    Cytotoxic Drugs   174
        Alkylating Agents   174
        Antimetabolites   175
        Antibiotics and Other Natural Products 176

Antibodies	178	
Other Cytotoxic Drugs	178	
Hormonal Agents	179	
Kinase Inhibitors	180	
Miscellaneous Agents	180	

PART **VI**

DRUGS THAT AFFECT THE ENDOCRINE SYSTEM

36. ADRENOCORTICAL HORMONES	185
Organization of Class	185
Glucocorticoids	187
Mineralocorticoids	188
Inhibitors of Adrenocorticoid Synthesis	188
37. SEX STEROIDS	189
Organization of Class	189
Estrogens	191
Antiestrogens	191
Progestins	192
Antiprogestins	192
Oral Contraceptives	192
Androgens	193
Antiandrogens	194
GnRH Agonists and Antagonists	194
PDE5 Inhibitors	195
38. THYROID AND PARATHYROID DRUGS	196
Organization of Class	196
Thyroid Replacement Therapy	197
Drugs That Are Thyroid Downers	197
Parathyroid Drugs	197
39. INSULIN, GLUCAGON, AND ORAL HYPOGLYCEMIC DRUGS	199
Organization of Class	199
Insulins	200
Oral Hypoglycemic Agents	201

PART **VII**

MISCELLANEOUS DRUGS

40. HISTAMINE AND ANTIHISTAMINES	205
Organization of Class	205
H_1 Receptor Antagonists	205
41. RESPIRATORY DRUGS	208
Organization of Class	208
β-Agonists	209
Leukotriene Modifiers	209
Methylxanthines	210
Cholinergic Antagonists	210
Cromolyn and Omalizumab	210
Pulmonary Hypertension	210
42. DRUGS THAT AFFECT THE GI TRACT	212
Organization of Class	212
Drugs That Act in the Upper GI Tract	212
Drugs That Act in the Lower GI Tract	213
43. NONNARCOTIC ANALGESICS AND ANTI-INFLAMMATORY DRUGS	216
Organization of Class	216
Nonsteroidal Anti-Inflammatory Drugs	216
Cox-2 Inhibitors	218
Salicylates, Including Aspirin	218
Acetaminophen	220
Other Drugs for Arthritis	220
Antigout Agents	221
Drugs Used in the Treatment of Headaches	222
44. IMMUNOSUPPRESSIVES	223
Organization of Class	223
Calcineurin Inhibitors	223
Mycophenolate Mofetil and Azathioprine	224
Monoclonal Antibodies	224
45. DRUGS USED IN OSTEOPOROSIS	225
Organization of Class	225
Bisphosphonates	226
Selective Estrogen Receptor Modulators	226
Estrogens	226
Parathyroid Hormone	227
Calcitonin	227
Other Agents	227
46. TOXICOLOGY AND POISONING	228
Principles of Toxicology	228
General Principles in the Treatment of Poisoning	228
Specific Antidotes	229
Index	231

Preface

Basic Concepts in Pharmacology: What You Need to Know for Each Drug Class is not a conventional review book for pharmacology. It is a book to help you organize your attack on the hundreds of drugs covered in pharmacology classes today. It is hoped that using this book will minimize the stress resulting from just thinking about all those drugs. Our survey for the first edition of this book made it clear that it is the number of drugs in a particular class that students find overwhelming. This fear causes many students to lose focus on the most important part of pharmacology—the concepts.

Because this is not a review book, I will not be covering each and every drug currently available. Instead, I will try to provide a way to organize and condense the amount of material that needs to be memorized. In addition, certain concepts and definitions will be explained. Along the way we will need to review some biochemistry and physiology, reinforcing previously learned concepts.

This book is organized so that the reader can read the highlights and decide whether or not to read the more detailed description.

Once you understand the material, you need not waste your time with the explanation. This book is intended to help you organize your study and avoid any extra hours spent on less important trivia, so you should approach the book in the same way.

Some drug names appear in capital letters. Although somewhat of an arbitrary choice, these drug names seem to be the most important to know. If you have time and energy to learn only three names in a particular drug class, learn the ones that appear in capital letters. Because students are expected to know only generic names of drugs, only generic names are used throughout this text. Trade names are given in the index.

Information in the boxes is key. If you know the information in the box, skip to the next one. If you don't know the information, read the text that follows it.

Where to Start

You cannot possibly learn everything about every drug available. Although many pharmacology students are able to memorize an incredible amount of useful and useless information, there is a limit to what even the best students can learn. Therefore, you must try to organize the material in a way that minimizes the amount of information you have to memorize. You need to get the most bang for your buck, or most facts learned for each hour of time spent. Usually this means grouping drugs and making associations.

> The best approach is to learn drugs by their class.

New drugs will be introduced during your lifetime and even during your training, so it is necessary to develop a flexible framework for drug information.

Many students try to memorize everything about a drug and end up remembering the most trivial facts and forgetting the most important ones. From a student's perspective it is often very difficult to know what is a priority and what can be skipped. Textbooks are usually not helpful in guiding students in making these decisions because of the way they are organized. They give general information about the pathophysiology or the drug class, followed by details about each individual agent in the class. This is an efficient way to be thorough, and it is very useful when you need to go back and look up a detail about a drug. It is not, however, as useful for the beginning student who must start from scratch to learn the information.

To help you decide what is the most important information, I have developed a trivia sorter.

Trivia Sorter: Generic

1. The mechanism of action for the class of drug.

2. Properties or effects that are common to all drugs in the class.

3. Is (are) the drug(s) the *drug of choice* for some disorder or symptom?

4. Name recognition—what drugs are in this class?

5. Unique features about single drugs in the class.

6. Are there any side effects (rare or not) that may be *fatal?*

7. Drug interactions.

8. Rare side effects or actions that are common to all drugs in the class.

(Continued)

Trivia Sorter: Generic (*Continued*)

9. Rare side effects or actions for single drugs in the class.

10. Percentage of drug that is metabolized versus renal excretion.

11. Half-life of each drug in the class.

12. Teratogenicity of each drug in the class.

13. Structure of each drug in the class.

This generic trivia sorter will not work for all drug classes. Therefore, for each class I will indicate the way I have organized the attack on the drugs in that group. For example, the mechanism of action of the antiepileptic drugs is not clear, so you will have to skip step 1 and go to step 2. The antiarrhythmic agents are classified and grouped according to their mechanism of action, so that should be the number 1 item you learn.

You can determine your own trivia level. I would suggest at least through number 6. If you have the time and inclination to learn more details you will need to consult your favorite textbook.

Because the *drug of choice* is often very important to know, these drugs are included in the boxes that appear throughout the book. However, these are subject to change, so you should confirm that the drug is still the drug of choice during class or from your textbook. Fatal side effects, even if rare, are important to know for your patients' safety. I will try to point out some, but others may come up in class or in your textbook. If so, make a note to learn them.

Name recognition is a slightly different matter. From my own experience as well as that of many medical students, examination questions about unfamiliar drugs are usually skipped or answered incorrectly. However, if the drug class is identified, the question becomes simple. I recommend to students who are having trouble with drug name recognition to make flash cards (or lists) with only the drug name on one side and the drug class on the other side. Skip the easy ones. Quiz yourself during breakfast or during breaks between classes. As you learn the drugs take them off your list or remove the card from the stack. Occasionally put these names back and review all together. If you only get a few more questions right on an examination or on the boards, or have to look up one less drug after rounds, the few minutes that this takes will have been worth it.

PART I General Principles

CHAPTER 2: Receptor Theory 05

CHAPTER 3: Absorption, Distribution, and Clearance 11

CHAPTER 4: Pharmacokinetics 16

CHAPTER 5: Drug Metabolism and Renal Elimination 24

Receptor Theory

Agonists
Efficacy and Potency
Therapeutic Index
Antagonists
Inverse Agonists

AGONISTS

A drug receptor is a specialized target macromolecule that binds a drug and mediates its pharmacological action. These receptors may be enzymes, nucleic acids, or specialized membrane-bound proteins. The formation of the drug-receptor complex leads to a biological response. The magnitude of the response is proportional to the number of drug-receptor complexes. A common way to present the relationship between the drug concentration and the biological response is with a concentration- (or dose-) response curve (Figure 2–1). In many textbooks, you will see both dose-response curves and concentration-response curves. Because the biological effect is more closely related to the plasma concentration than to the dose, I will show concentration-response curves in this chapter.

> An agonist is a compound that binds to a receptor and produces the biological response.

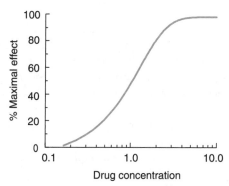

FIGURE 2–1 In a concentration-response curve, the concentration of the drug is plotted against the percent maximal effect. Notice that the drug concentration is plotted on a log scale. In this graph, the drug is a full agonist—the effect reaches 100% of the maximum possible.

An agonist can be a drug or the endogenous ligand for the receptor. Increasing concentrations of the agonist will increase the biological response until there are no more receptors for the agonist to bind or a maximal response has been reached.

> A partial agonist produces the biological response but cannot produce 100% of the biological response even at very high doses.

Partial agonists compared to "full" agonists (Figure 2–2).

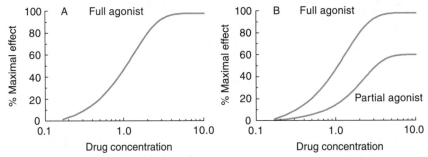

FIGURE 2–2 In A, the concentration-response curve for a full agonist is presented. The drug can produce a maximal effect. In B, the concentration-response curve for a partial agonist is also shown. In this case, the partial agonist is able to produce only 60% of the maximal response.

EFFICACY AND POTENCY

Efficacy and *potency* are terms that students sometimes confuse. These terms are used for comparisons between drugs.

> Efficacy is the maximal response a drug can produce. Potency is a measure of the dose that is required to produce a response.

For example, one drug (drug A) produces complete eradication of premature ventricular contractions (PVCs) at a dose of 10 mg. A second drug (drug B) produces complete eradication of PVCs at a dose of 20 mg. Therefore, both drugs have the same efficacy (complete eradication of PVCs), but drug A is more potent than drug B. It takes less of drug A to produce the same effect. A third drug (drug C) can reduce the PVCs by only 60%, and it takes a dose of 50 mg to achieve that effect. Therefore, drug C has less efficacy and less potency in the reduction of PVCs compared with both drug A and drug B.

Potency and efficacy are usually shown graphically (Figure 2–3).

> Potency is often expressed as the dose of a drug required to achieve 50% of the desired therapeutic effect. This is the ED_{50} (effective dose).

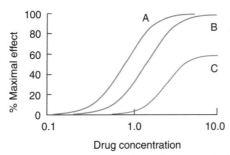

FIGURE 2–3 Concentration-response curves for drugs A, B, and C are presented. Drugs A and B have equal efficacy, but drug A is more potent than drug B. Drug C is less efficacious and less potent than either drug A or drug B.

THERAPEUTIC INDEX

Therapeutic index is a measure of drug safety. A drug with a higher therapeutic index is safer than one with a lower therapeutic index.

That statement is true no matter what textbook you consult. However, the definition of therapeutic index may vary depending on the book. Usually,

$$\text{Therapeutic index} = \frac{\text{LD}_{50}}{\text{ED}_{50}}$$

The lethal dose (LD_{50}) is the dose that kills 50% of the animals that receive it. Sometimes the TD_{50} is used in place of the LD_{50}. The TD_{50} is the dose that is toxic in 50% of the animals that receive it. Death is the ultimate toxicity.

The therapeutic index is sometimes confused with the therapeutic window. The therapeutic window is the range of plasma concentrations of a drug that will elicit the desired response in a population of patients.

ANTAGONISTS

Antagonists block or reverse the effect of agonists. They have no effect of their own.

Binding of an antagonist to a receptor does not produce a biological effect. The antagonist can block the effect of an agonist or it can reverse the effect of an agonist. An example of an antagonist is naloxone, an opioid antagonist (see Chapter 22). Naloxone has no effect of its own but will completely reverse the effects of any opioid agonist that has been administered. Sometimes the antagonist reverses or blocks the effect of endogenously produced compounds, such as epinephrine or norepinephrine. This is the mechanism of action of β-blockers.

> Competitive antagonists make the agonist look less potent by shifting the dose response curve to the right.

Because the antagonists theoretically have no effect of their own, we need to consider their effect on the agonist. In the graph in Figure 2–4, we determined the biological effect produced by a series of concentrations of agonist. We then repeat the same experiment in the presence of a fixed concentration of an antagonist. This shifts the curve to the right, making the agonist look less potent.

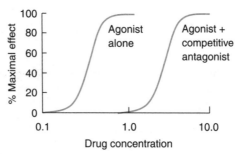

FIGURE 2–4 In this graph the concentration-response curve for an agonist alone is presented. When the effect of the agonist is tested in the presence of a fixed concentration of a competitive antagonist, the agonist appears less potent. The same maximal effect is achieved, but it takes higher doses to do so.

This is easy to remember and understand. These antagonists are competitive; that is, they compete for the same site on the receptor that the agonist wants. If the agonist wins, a response is produced. If the antagonist wins, no response is produced. As we increase the concentration of agonist, we increase the odds that an agonist molecule will win the receptor spot and produce an effect. At a high enough agonist concentration, the poor antagonist doesn't have a chance at the receptor; it is simply outnumbered.

> A noncompetitive antagonist reduces the maximal response that an agonist can produce.

Let's repeat the earlier experiment. We first determine the biological effect produced by increasing concentrations of an agonist. We repeat these measurements in the presence of a fixed concentration of a noncompetitive antagonist (Figure 2–5). Increasing concentrations of the agonist cannot overcome this blockade. Therefore, the maximal biological response produced by the agonist appears to have decreased because of our addition of the noncompetitive antagonist.

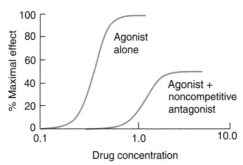

FIGURE 2–5 The concentration-response curve for the same agonist alone is presented. Then the activity of the agonist is tested in the presence of a fixed concentration of noncompetitive antagonist. In this instance the maximal response is reduced.

There are a number of molecular mechanisms by which noncompetitive antagonists can reduce the maximal effect. They can irreversibly bind to the receptor so that the agonist cannot be competed off, they can bind to a site different from the agonist and either prevent agonist binding or prevent the agonist effect. Some books will use different terminology, such as uncompetitive, for the different mechanisms.

INVERSE AGONISTS

> Inverse agonists have opposite effects from those of full agonists. They are not the same as antagonists, which block the effects of both agonists and inverse agonists.

The term *inverse agonist* has been around for a number of years. Originally, it was used to describe the action of some drugs on conductance through ligand-gated ion channels. Most ion channels have a basal rate of opening and closing. Agonsts will increase the relative amount of time the channel is in the open state compared to the basal rate. Inverse agonists will decrease the amount of time the channel is open compared to the basal rate. At the $GABA_A$ receptor channel complex, agonists increase the amount of chloride that moves into the neuron and will hyperpolarize it. Overall, this leads to sedation. An inverse agonist will decrease the amount of chloride that moves into the neuron, which will result in a depolarization compared to the resting state. Overall, this leads to an increase in excitability and can cause seizures.

We now know that a number of G protein–coupled receptors have basal activity. Current theory states that G protein–coupled receptors are in an equilibrium between an active and inactive state. Inverse agonists bind to the receptor and tip the equilibrium toward the inactive state, while agonists bind the receptor and tip the equilibrium toward the active state. For there to be inverse agonist in a receptor system, there must be activity in the basal, resting state in the absence of any ligand.

While the net physiological result of giving an inverse agonist and an antagonist may be the same, the molecular mechanism is not. Antagonists bind to the receptor, but they have no effect on the basal state. They do, however, block the effects of both the agonists and inverse agonists (Figure 2–6).

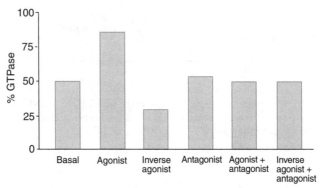

FIGURE 2–6 This graph illustrates the concept of an inverse agonist. Basal GTPase activity is compared with activity in the presence of an agonist and an inverse agonist. An antagonist has no effect on GTPase activity and completely blocks the effects of both the agonist and inverse agonist.

Absorption, Distribution, and Clearance

First-Pass Effect
How Drugs Cross Membranes
Bioavailability
Total Body Clearance

FIRST-PASS EFFECT

> The liver is a metabolic machine and often inactivates drugs on their way from the GI tract to the body. This is called the first-pass effect.

Orally administered drugs are absorbed from the gastrointestinal (GI) tract. The blood from the GI tract then travels through the liver, the great chemical plant in the body. Many drugs that undergo liver metabolism will be extensively metabolized during this passage from the GI tract to the body. This effect of liver metabolism is called the first-pass effect.

HOW DRUGS CROSS MEMBRANES

There are several useful routes of drug administration, but almost all require that the drug cross a biological membrane to reach its site of action.

> Drugs cross membranes by passive diffusion or active transport.

This statement is somewhat simplified, but it provides a useful starting point. Passive diffusion requires a concentration gradient across the membrane. The vast majority of drugs gain access to their site of action by this method. Water-soluble drugs can penetrate the cell membrane through aqueous channels. More commonly lipid-soluble drugs just move through the membrane.

> A drug tends to pass through membranes if it is uncharged.

Uncharged drugs are more lipid soluble than charged drugs. In addition, many drugs are weak acids or weak bases.

> For a weak acid, when the pH is less than the pK, the protonated form (nonionized) predominates. When the pH is greater than the pK, the unprotonated (ionized) form predominates.

$$HA \leftrightarrows H^+ + A^-$$

Weak acids are hydrogen ion donors; they are happy to give up a hydrogen ion and become charged. If you have trouble remembering whether they become charged or uncharged after donating their hydrogen ion, think of a strong acid, such as HCl. As you know, when you put HCl into water it immediately turns into H^+ and Cl^-. Use this example to remember that weak acids donate a hydrogen ion and become charged.

Remember the pK? That is the equilibrium constant (of course, the p means we've taken the negative log of the equilibrium constant). When the pH is equal to the pK, the preceding equation is balanced. There are equal amounts of weak acid in the ionized and nonionized forms. If we decrease the pH by adding more H^+, we will drive the equilibrium for the weak acid more to the left, which is the nonionized (uncharged) form.

If we take away H^+, making the pH higher, we will drive the equilibrium toward the right. This increases the concentration of the ionized form of the weak acid (Figure 3–1).

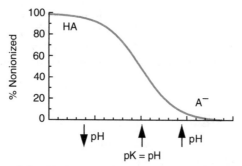

FIGURE 3-1 The relationship between the pH and the degree of ionization of a weak acid is presented. When the pH is higher than the pK for the acid, the charged form of the acid predominates.

> For a weak base, when the pH is less than the pK, the ionized form (protonated) predominates. When the pH is greater than the pK, the unprotonated (nonionized) form predominates.

Weak bases are the opposite of weak acids. A weak base is a hydrogen ion acceptor. If a loose hydrogen ion seeks to join it, the base may accept it. If it accepts the hydrogen ion, then it becomes charged.

$$B + H^+ \leftrightarrows BH^+$$

Adding H^+ to lower the pH will drive the equilibrium to the right toward the protonated (charged) form. Removing H^+ to raise the pH will drive the equilibrium to the left toward the uncharged form (unprotonated) of the base (Figure 3–2).

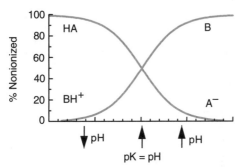

FIGURE 3–2 In this graph the effects of pH on the degree of ionization of both a weak acid and a weak base are presented.

> In the stomach (pH 2.0), weak acids are uncharged and will be absorbed into the bloodstream, whereas weak bases are charged and will remain in the GI tract.

To test your understanding of this, try out these questions. Answers appear at the bottom of the page.*

1. In the intestine (pH 8.0), which will be better absorbed, a weak acid (pK 6.8) or a weak base (pK 7.1)?

2. If we alkalinize the urine to a pH of 7.8, will a lower or higher percentage of a weak acid (pK 7.1) be ionized, compared with when the urine pH was 7.2?

BIOAVAILABILITY

> *Bioavailability* is the amount of drug that is absorbed after administration by route X compared with the amount of drug that is absorbed after intravenous (IV) administration. X is any route of drug administration other than IV.

Example: Suppose you are testing a compound in clinical trials. You have tentatively named this compound "Newdrug." Newdrug is administered orally and plasma levels determine that only 75% of the oral dose reaches the circulation.

*Answers: (1) a weak base; (2) higher, because more weak acid will be ionized the more the pH exceeds the pK.

Compared with intravenous (IV) administration where 100% of the dose reaches the circulation, the bioavailability of Newdrug is 0.75 or 75%. In the case of hypothetical Newdrug, you discover that some of the drug is inactivated by the acid in the stomach. You redesign the pill with a coating that is stable in acid but dissolves in the more basic pH of the small intestine. The bioavailability of the drug increases to 95%. Newdrug becomes a best-selling product(Figure 3–3).

$$Bioavailability = \frac{AUC_{oral}}{AUC_{IV}}$$

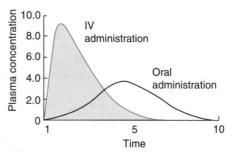

FIGURE 3–3 The plasma concentration plotted against the time and the area under the curve (AUC) is an indication of bioavailability. In this graph, an orally administered drug is compared with the same drug administered intravenously.

TOTAL BODY CLEARANCE

Clearance is a term that indicates the rate at which a drug is cleared from the body. It is defined as the volume of plasma from which all drug is removed in a given time. Thus, the units for clearance are given in volume per unit time.

Clearance is an odd term, mostly because of the units used to report it. It is not intuitive. Try the following exercise as a way to remember the units.

Suppose we have a 10-L aquarium that contains 10,000 mg of crud. The concentration is 1 mg/mL. Clearance is 1 L/h. In other words, the aquarium filter and pump clear 1 L of water in an hour. At the end of the first hour, 1000 mg of crud has been removed from the aquarium (1000 mL of 1 mg/mL). The aquarium thus has 9000 mg of crud remaining, for a concentration of 0.9 mg/mL. At the end of the second hour, 900 mg of crud has been removed (1000 mL of 0.9 mg/mL). The aquarium now has 8100 mg of crud remaining, for a concentration of 0.81 mg/mL. This process continues forever. Notice that the time to clear this particular aquarium is not 10 hours. It would take 10 hours (10 L at 1 L/h) if the clean water was pumped into another container. In the case of clearance in the aquarium, however, the clean water is returned to the tank and dilutes the remaining crud (Figure 3–4). The same principle holds true for clearance of a drug from the human body.

Pump filter rate = clearance

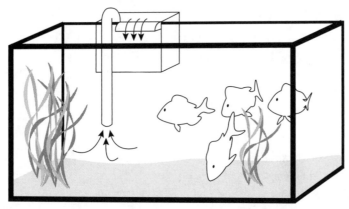

FIGURE 3-4 Clearance is very much like an aquarium pump. The pump cleans a fixed amount of water in the aquarium in a set amount of time (the clearance). The clean water returns to the aquarium, diluting the remaining water.

A more official definition is the following equation:

$$\text{Clearance} = \frac{\text{Rate of removal of drug (mg/min)}}{\text{Plasma concentration of drug (mg/min)}}$$

Notice that this equation gives you units of milliliters per minute (mL/min) or volume per unit time.

Total body clearance is the sum of the clearances from the various organs involved in drug metabolism and elimination.

4

Pharmacokinetics

Volume of Distribution
First-Order Kinetics
Zero-Order Kinetics
Steady-State Concentration
Time Needed to Reach Steady State
Loading Dose

Pharmacokinetics is the mathematical description of the rate and extent of uptake, distribution, and elimination of drugs in the body.

VOLUME OF DISTRIBUTION

Volume of distribution (V_D) is a calculation of the apparent volume in which a drug is dissolved. It assumes that a drug is evenly distributed and that metabolism or elimination has not taken place. In reality, it does not correspond to any real volume:

$$\text{Volume of distribution}\,(V_D) = \frac{\text{Dose (mg)}}{\text{Plasma concentration (mg/mL)}}$$

This equation is very easy to remember. Suppose you take 1000 mg of sugar and dissolve it into a beaker of water. After it has dissolved, you take a sample of water (let's say, 10 mL) and determine the concentration of sugar in that sample (for example, 1 mg/mL). From this finding you can calculate the volume of water in which the sugar was dissolved, as follows:

$$1 \text{ mg/mL} = 1000 \text{ mg/volume of water}$$

thus,

$$\text{Volume} = \frac{1000 \text{ mg}}{1 \text{ mg/mL}} = 1000 \text{ mL}$$

In this case the volume was 1000 mL or 1 L. If you keep the units straight, the equation does not need to be memorized.

Try another one. Suppose 500 mg of "Newdrug" is administered to a medical student. The plasma concentration is 0.01 mg/mL. What is the volume of distribution?*

The volume of distribution is rather large. Your selected medical student is not, however, a huge water balloon. The only explanation is that the drug is hiding someplace in the body where it is not recorded by the measurement of plasma concentration. The drug could be lipid soluble and stored in fat, or it could be bound to plasma proteins. As this example shows, the volume of distribution is a hypothetical volume and not a real volume.

The volume of distribution gives a rough accounting of where a drug goes in the body, especially if you have a feel for the various body fluid compartments and their sizes (Figure 4–1). In addition, it can be used to calculate the dose of a drug needed to achieve a desired plasma concentration.

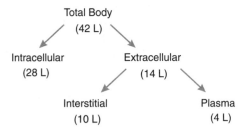

FIGURE 4–1 The various body fluid compartments for a standard 70-kg man are illustrated in this figure.

FIRST-ORDER KINETICS

The order of a reaction refers to the way in which the concentration of drug or reactant influences the rate of a chemical reaction. For most drugs, we need only consider first-order and zero-order.

> Most drugs disappear from plasma by processes that are concentration-dependent, which results in first-order kinetics. With first-order elimination, a constant percentage of the drug is lost per unit time. An elimination rate constant can be described.

The elimination rate constant is k_e (units are 1/time). On the log plot (Figure 4–2), the curve is linear and the slope of the line is equal to $k_e/2.303$. The factor 2.303 converts from natural log to base 10 log units.

> The half-life ($t_{1/2}$) is the period of time required for the concentration of a drug to decrease by one half.

---

*Answer: 50,000 mL or 50 L.

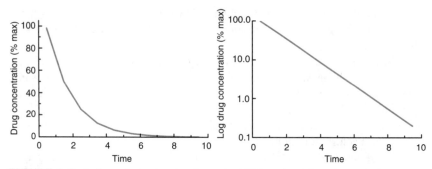

FIGURE 4–2 Both graphs present the elimination of a drug that follows first-order kinetics. On the left, the y-axis is a linear scale, while on the right, the y-axis is a logarithmic scale. Notice that first-order reactions are linear when graphed on the log scale.

The half-life, or $t_{1/2}$, is shown graphically in Figure 4–3.

> The half-life is constant and related to k_e for drugs that have first-order kinetics.
>
> $$t_{1/2} = 0.693/k_e$$

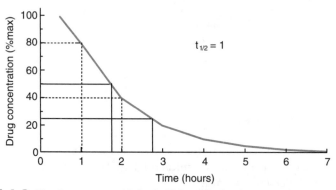

FIGURE 4–3 The determination of the half-life ($t_{1/2}$) of a drug with first-order kinetics is illustrated. The drug concentration is graphed against the time. The time it takes for the concentration to decrease by 50% is indicated in two places on the curve. The $t_{1/2}$ is the same for both determinations.

First-order elimination rate

= rate constant × plasma concentration × volume of distribution

= $k(1/\text{min}) \times C_p(\text{mg/mL}) \times V_D(\text{mL})$

= mg/min

> Clearance of a drug is different from the elimination rate.

Remember clearance? As explained in Chapter 3, it's the volume of fluid cleared of a drug per unit time. In contrast, the elimination rate is the rate of removal of drug in weight per unit time. For drugs with first-order kinetics, clearance and elimination rate are related, as shown in the following equation:

$$\text{Clearance} = \frac{\text{Rate of removal of drug (mg/min)}}{\text{Plasma concentration of drug (mg/mL)}}$$

For drugs with first-order kinetics, the V_D, $t_{1/2}$, k_e, and clearance are all interrelated.

ZERO-ORDER KINETICS

Drugs that saturate routes of elimination disappear from plasma in a non–concentration-dependent manner, which is zero-order kinetics.

Metabolism in the liver, which involves specific enzymes, is one of the most important factors that contribute to a drug having zero-order kinetics. The most common examples of drugs that have zero-order kinetics are aspirin, phenytoin, and ethanol. Many drugs will show zero-order kinetics at high, or toxic, concentrations.

For drugs with zero-order kinetics, a constant amount of drug is lost per unit time. The half-life is not constant for zero-order reactions, but depends on the concentration.

The higher the concentration, the longer the $t_{1/2}$. This is illustrated in Figure 4–4. Because the $t_{1/2}$ changes as the drug concentration declines, the zero-order $t_{1/2}$ has little practical significance.

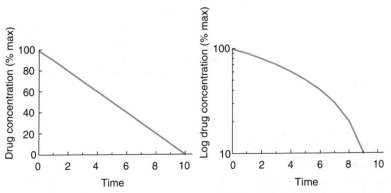

FIGURE 4–4 A drug showing zero-order elimination kinetics is illustrated here. On the left, the drug concentration is plotted on a linear scale and on the right, on a logarithmic scale. Notice that drugs with zero-order kinetics show a straight line on the linear scale. Try calculating the half-life of this drug in at least two different places. Do you get the same value?

Zero-order kinetics is also known as nonlinear or dose-dependent kinetics.

You will see the terms *zero-order, nonlinear,* and *dose-dependent* used interchangeably in the medical literature. The term *dose-dependent* refers to drugs that are first-order at lower doses and switch to zero-order at higher doses (often in the therapeutic range). Therefore, the kinetics of these drugs are dose-dependent. *Nonlinear* refers to the fact that drugs with zero-order kinetics do not show a linear relationship between drug dose and plasma concentration.

STEADY-STATE CONCENTRATION

> With multiple dosing, or a continuous infusion, a drug will accumulate until the amount administered per unit time is equal to the amount eliminated per unit time. The plasma concentration at this point is called the steady-state concentration (C_{ss}).

Rarely are drugs given as a single dose. Normally repeated doses are given and sometimes drugs are given as a continuous intravenous (IV) infusion. When a drug is given as a continuous infusion it will increase in concentration in the blood until the rate of elimination is equal to the infusion rate. At this point the amount going in per unit time is equal to the amount going out. The plasma concentration at this point is called the concentration at steady state, or C_{ss} (Figure 4–5).

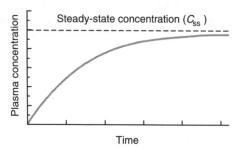

FIGURE 4–5 A continuous IV infusion of a drug was started at the beginning point of the graph. The concentration of the drug in the plasma was followed over time. When the amount delivered in a unit of time is equal to the amount eliminated in the same time unit, the plasma concentration is said to have reached steady state.

Let's consider a patient who has no drug in his system. You start an IV infusion at 100 mg/kg. At first the plasma level will be low and the infusion rate will be greater than the elimination rate. The plasma level will rise relatively quickly. Remember that the elimination rate is proportional to the plasma concentration of the drug, so as the concentration rises so does the elimination rate. As the elimination rate increases with the increasing plasma concentration, the rate of increase in the plasma level will slow. At steady state, the infusion rate and the elimination rate are equal.

For an IV infusion,

$$C_{ss} = \frac{\text{Infusion rate (mg/min)}}{\text{Clearance (mL/min)}} = \text{mg/mL}$$

Notice the direct relationship between C_{ss} and the infusion rate (assuming clearance is constant). If we double the infusion rate, the C_{ss} doubles.

There is also a concentration at steady state for repeated doses. Some textbooks call this an average concentration (C_{av}). With multiple dosing schedules, we normally assume that early doses of the drug do not affect the pharmacokinetics of subsequent doses. Generally, we also give equal doses at equal time intervals.

> Repeated dosing is associated with peak and trough plasma concentrations.

With repeated dosing the concentration fluctuates around a mean (steady-state value) with peak and trough values. Here, steady state is achieved when the dose administered and the amount eliminated in a given dosing interval is the same (Figure 4–6). The goal is to have the concentration remain within the therapeutic window, where it is effective, but not toxic. Sometimes this is not the case with a chosen dosing schedule. Either the peak reaches into the toxic range, in which case the patient experiences side effects, or the trough drops too low and the drug is no longer effective. Both of these problems can be solved by adjusting the dose and dosing schedule.

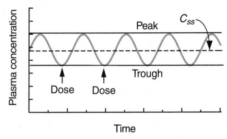

FIGURE 4–6 This graph shows the change in concentration with repeated doses. Peak and trough levels are indicated, as well as the steady-state concentration (or average concentration).

TIME NEEDED TO REACH STEADY STATE

So far we've focused on the concentration at steady state. Now let's consider the time it takes to reach this steady-state concentration.

> The time needed to reach steady state depends only on the half-life of the drug. Ninety percent of steady state is reached in 3.3 half-lives.

There is a good bit of math behind these numbers, which you can read about elsewhere if you want. The bottom line is that during each half-life, 50% of the change from the starting point to C_{ss} is achieved.

After one half-life, we gain 50% of the C_{ss}. We have 50% of the distance remaining. In the next half-life, we will gain 50% of this remaining distance, or 1/2 of 50%, which is 25%. So, after two half-lives, we will be 75% of the way to steady state. If you repeat this several times, you can generate the Table 4–1. Notice that after five half-lives, we are still approaching steady state.

TABLE 4–1   Percentage of Steady State (C_{ss}) Achieved after Every Half-Live ($t_{1/2}$)

No. of $t_{1/2}$	% C_{ss}
1	50
2	75
3	88
3.3	90
4	94
5	97

When asked the question, how long does it take to get to steady state, some sources accept 3.3 half-lives (90% of C_{ss}), whereas others use 4 half-lives (94% of C_{ss}), and still others accept 5 half-lives (97% of C_{ss}). Check your textbook or lecture notes.

LOADING DOSE

If the half-life of a drug is relatively long, such as ~6 days for digitoxin, it will take quite a long time for the drug concentration to reach steady state (about four times the half-life). For digitoxin, this would take over 3 weeks. Sometimes the patient can't wait that long for the therapeutic effect to occur. In these instances a loading dose is used.

> A loading dose is a single large dose of a drug that is used to raise the plasma concentration to a therapeutic level more quickly than would occur through repeated smaller doses.

A single dose of a drug can be given that will result in the desired plasma concentration. This dose is called a loading dose if followed by repeated doses or a continuous infusion that will maintain the plasma concentration at the desired level (termed maintenance doses).

As you can see in Figure 4–7, as the concentration begins to decline after the loading dose, the concentration contributed by the continuous infusion begins to increase.

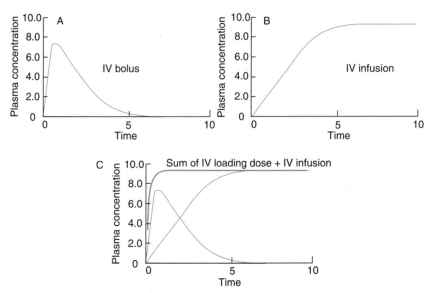

FIGURE 4–7 In A, the change in drug concentration as a function of time after an IV bolus is presented. In B, the change in drug concentration as a function of time after the start of a continuous IV infusion is presented. In C, both the bolus and the continuous infusion are given at time 0. The IV bolus is the loading dose. Notice how quickly the plasma concentration reaches the steady-state concentration with this technique.

5 Drug Metabolism and Renal Elimination

Liver Metabolism

Renal Excretion

LIVER METABOLISM

The liver is the major site for drug metabolism. The goal of metabolism is to produce metabolites that are polar, or charged, and can be eliminated by the kidney. Lipid-soluble agents are metabolized by the liver using two general sets of reactions, called phase I and phase II.

> Phase I reactions frequently involve the P-450 system. Phase II reactions are conjugations, mostly with glucuronide.

Phase I reactions convert lipophilic molecules into more polar molecules by introducing or unmasking a polar functional group, such as an —OH or —NH$_2$. Most of these reactions utilize the microsomal P-450 enzymes.

Phase I reactions are the basis of a number of drug interactions. There are a whole series of cytochrome P-450 enzymes that can be inhibited or induced. Of these, CYP3A4 plays a role in the metabolism of about 50% of the drugs that are currently prescribed. Inhibition or induction of CYP3A4 by one drug will affect the levels of any other drug that is also metabolized by CYP3A4. For example, rifampin induces CYP3A4 which can increase metabolism of estrogen, thus reducing the effectiveness of birth control pills. Some textbooks include lists of drugs that inhibit or induce CYP3A4. Don't try to memorize these lists. Be aware of the potential problem and learn the most commonly interacting drugs as you gain experience. There are also known genetic variations in levels of CYP450 enzymes.

Phase II reactions are conjugation reactions. These combine a glucuronic acid, sulfuric acid, acetic acid, or an amino acid with the drug molecule to make it more polar. The highly polar drugs can then by excreted by the kidney.

RENAL EXCRETION

> Renal elimination of drugs involves three physiological processes: glomerular filtration, proximal tubular secretion, and distal tubular reabsorption.

1. *Glomerular filtration:* Free drug flows out of the body and into the urine-to-be as part of the glomerular filtrate. The size of the molecule is the only limiting factor at this step.

2. *Proximal tubular secretion:* Some drugs are actively secreted into the proximal tubule.

3. *Distal tubular reabsorption:* Uncharged drugs may diffuse out of the kidney and escape elimination. Manipulating the pH of the urine may alter this process by changing the ionization of the weak acids and bases. This process was described in Chapter 3 in the context of passive diffusion of drugs across membranes. However, for a drug to be excreted, it needs to be charged so that it is trapped in the urine and can't cross the membrane to sneak back into the body.

> **Reminder:** When the pH is higher than the pK, the unprotonated forms (A^- and B) predominate. When the pH is less than the pK, the protonated forms (HA and BH^+) predominate.

PART II Drugs That Affect the Autonomic Nervous System

CHAPTER 6: Review of the Autonomic Nervous System   29

CHAPTER 7: Cholinergic Agonists   38

CHAPTER 8: Cholinergic Antagonists   43

CHAPTER 9: Adrenergic Agonists   47

CHAPTER 10: Adrenergic Antagonists   52

Review of the Autonomic Nervous System

Why Include This Material?

Relevant Anatomy

Synthesis, Storage, Release, and Removal of Transmitters

Receptors

General Rules of Innervation

Presynaptic Receptors

WHY INCLUDE THIS MATERIAL?

Why include a review of the autonomic nervous system in a book on pharmacology? The main reason is that autonomic pharmacology is easiest if you have an understanding of the anatomy and physiology of the autonomic nervous system. Therefore, a quick review of the autonomic nervous system should simplify the pharmacology. In addition, autonomic pharmacology forms a basis for cardiovascular and central nervous system pharmacology. Consequently, learning the autonomics thoroughly will save you time and effort later on.

It is hoped that you learned the anatomy and physiology of the autonomic nervous system in your anatomy and physiology classes. Let's begin with a quiz to see how much you remember and then move on to a review of the pertinent facts.

Fill in the blanks in the following sentences. If you can do so easily, you are in great shape and should skip the rest of this chapter.*

1. All preganglionic fibers of the autonomic nervous system use the neurotransmitter _____.

2. The major neurotransmitter for sympathetic postganglionic fibers is _____.

3. Stimulation of sympathetic innervation to the eye causes contraction of the _____ muscle and, therefore, _____ of the pupil.

4. The rate-limiting step in the synthesis of norepinephrine is _____.

5. The major pathway for the termination of the action of norepinephrine is _____.

6. The actions of acetylcholine released from parasympathetic fibers in viscera are mediated by _____ receptors.

7. Adrenergic receptors in the heart are predominantly _____.

8. Stimulation of α_1 receptors causes predominantly _____of blood vessels.

9. Stimulation of the sympathetic nervous system causes _____in gluconeogenesis and glycogenolysis.

10. Stimulation of the β_2 receptor in the pregnant uterus causes _____ of the smooth muscle.

Some of the preceding sentences required you to supply information that is pretty picky. If you completed all of them correctly, you did great. If you completed most, you're doing really well. If you were only able to fill in a few of the blanks, please read on.

RELEVANT ANATOMY

The nervous system is divided into two main parts, the central nervous system and the peripheral nervous system (Figure 6–1). The central nervous system is made up of the brain and spinal cord. The peripheral nervous system contains everything else, including all of the sensory information going to the brain and all of the information flowing out of the brain. The peripheral nervous system is divided into two branches, the somatic and autonomic nervous systems. The somatic nervous system is mainly the motor system, which includes all of the nerves to the muscles. The other branch, the autonomic nervous system, is the part we're interested in here.

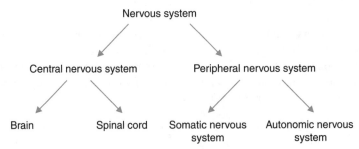

FIGURE 6–1 This diagram shows the major divisions of the nervous system.

> The autonomic nervous system is responsible for maintaining the internal environment of the body (homeostasis).

*Answers: (1) acetylcholine; (2) norepinephrine; (3) radial, dilation; (4) the formation of dopa by tyrosine β-hydroxylase; (5) reuptake; (6) muscarinic; (7) β_1; (8) constriction; (9) an increase; (10) relaxation.

Knowing the role of the autonomic nervous system in homeostasis makes it easy to remember the target organs served by this system. It is clear that the cardiovascular system needs regulation, but the smooth muscle of the gastrointestinal (GI) tract and the various glands throughout the body also need to be constantly monitored. Let's first consider some points that are true about the *entire* autonomic nervous system before we break the system down into parts.

> Within the autonomic nervous system, two neurons are required to reach a target organ, a preganglionic neuron and a postganglionic neuron.

The preganglionic neuron originates in the central nervous system. It forms a synapse with the postganglionic neuron, the cell body of which is located in autonomic ganglia. Simple enough.

> *All* preganglionic neurons release acetylcholine as their transmitter. The acetylcholine binds to nicotinic receptors on the postganglionic cell.

The preceding statement is a general rule. We'll come back to the transmitter and receptors in more detail later.

The autonomic nervous system is divided into the sympathetic and parasympathetic systems (Figure 6–2). The sympathetic system is catabolic, meaning that it burns energy. It is the one involved in the fight-or-flight response. If you remember this, most of the effects of the sympathetic nervous system make sense. The sympathetic nervous system is also called the thoracolumbar system because the ganglia are located lateral to the vertebral column in the thoracic and lumbar regions. In addition, because the ganglia are fixed along the back, the postganglionic fibers can be quite long. Within the sympathetic system the preganglionic axons form synapses with many postganglionic cells, thus giving this system a widespread action. Note that this is consistent with the fight-or-flight response.

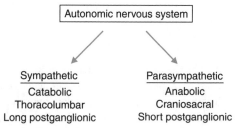

FIGURE 6–2 The two divisions of the autonomic nervous system are illustrated, along with some of the key features of each division.

The parasympathetic system is anabolic, meaning that it tries to conserve energy. It is sometimes called the craniosacral system. The preganglionic neurons are found in the brain stem and in the sacral region of the spinal cord. In the parasympathetic system, the ganglia are located closer to the target organs (they are not fixed along the vertebral column). Therefore, the preganglionic axons tend to be longer and the postganglionic fibers are shorter. Within the parasympathetic system, one presynaptic axon tends to form a synapse with only one or two postganglionic cells, giving the parasympathetic system a more localized action.

> *All* of the parasympathetic postganglionic fibers release acetylcholine. At the target organ acetylcholine interacts with muscarinic receptors.

The key word here is *all*. More on the muscarinic receptors later.

> *Most* of the sympathetic postganglionic fibers release norepinephrine. At the target organ norepinephrine interacts with a variety of receptors.

The key word here is *most*. Most of the sympathetic system utilizes norepinephrine (NE), but acetylcholine is also found (in sweat glands). In addition, the adrenal medulla is considered part of the sympathetic nervous system and it releases epinephrine (EPI) (80%) and NE. Note also that NE is equivalent to nor*adren*aline, and that EPI is equivalent to *adren*aline (hence the term *adren*ergic).

SYNTHESIS, STORAGE, RELEASE, AND REMOVAL OF TRANSMITTERS

The synthesis, storage, release, and removal of transmitters is important because there are drugs that target each of these steps. It is not really necessary to memorize the complete pathway for synthesis of every neurotransmitter; however, a few points are important. Let's start with acetylcholine.

> Acetylcholine is synthesized from acetyl coenzyme A (acetyl CoA) and choline. Its action is terminated by acetylcholinesterase.

It is easy to remember the precursors of acetylcholine from the spelling of its name. Notice that *acetyl* CoA plus *choline* gives you acetylcholine. Likewise, the ending "-esterase" identifies the enzyme that breaks down the acetylcholine.

Now let's turn to NE and its close relative, EPI. It is important to know the pathway for synthesis of these two compounds, at least by name (Figure 6–3). You might also try to remember the details of the biochemistry if you have time.

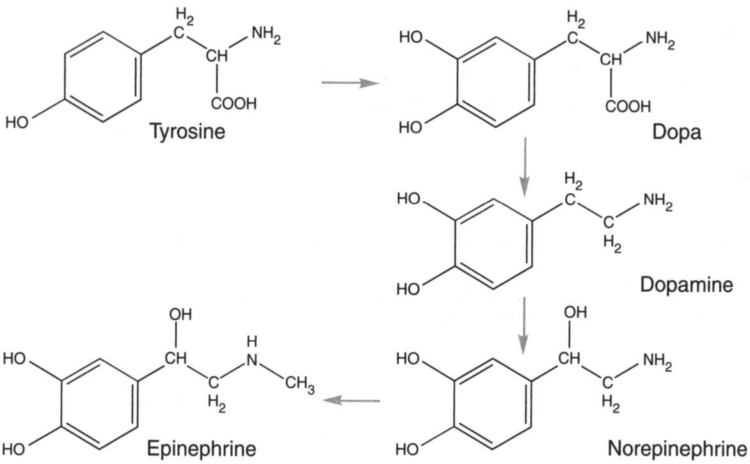

FIGURE 6–3 The synthesis of NE and EPI is illustrated. Note the close relationship between dopamine, NE, and EPI.

The rate-limiting step in the synthesis of NE and EPI is the conversion of tyrosine to dopa by tyrosine β-hydroxylase. Although this step is not very important pharmacologically, it seems to appear as an examination question in rather unpredictable places.

> The effect of NE is terminated predominantly by reuptake into the neuron from which it was released.

Norepinephrine can also be inactivated by enzymes in the liver (mostly) and brain (some). The degradative enzymes are called COMT (catechol-o-methyltransferase) and MAO (monoamine oxidase). MAO comes in two forms, A and B. COMT, particularly in the liver, plays a major role in the metabolism of endogenously released (circulating) and exogenously administered EPI and NE.

Note: You will often hear the term *catecholamine*. This refers to the structure of this group of compounds. They have a catechol group and an amine group, as shown in Figure 6–4.

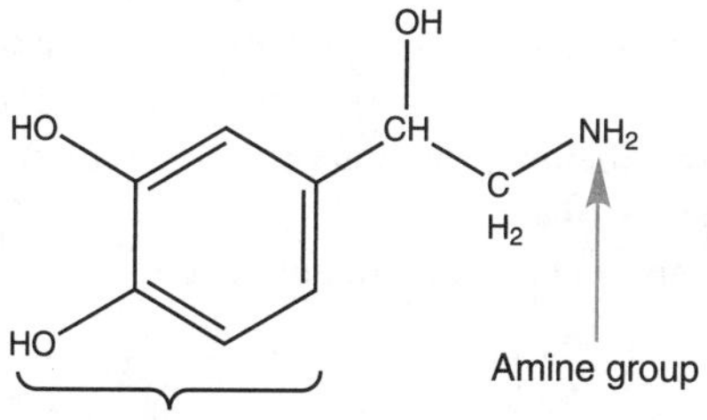

FIGURE 6–4 The general catecholamine structure is illustrated. The catechol group consists of a benzene ring with two hydroxyl groups.

RECEPTORS

At this point, you probably know that there are classes of receptors for neurotransmitters. Each class is further broken down into subtypes. For the big picture, don't worry about the subtypes for now. For simplicity's sake, let's first consider the receptors for acetylcholine.

> There are two major classes of receptors for acetylcholine, muscarinic and nicotinic (Figure 6–5).

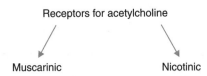

FIGURE 6–5   The types of acetylcholine receptors are illustrated.

There are subtypes of muscarinic receptors (M_1, M_2, and so on), and there are at least two types of nicotinic receptors. Don't attempt to memorize these subtypes until you understand the bigger picture.

> *All* of the parasympathetic postganglionic fibers release acetylcholine. At the target organ the acetylcholine interacts with muscarinic receptors.

This information should look familiar, because the same statement was highlighted in an earlier box. These muscarinic receptors are predominantly found in the viscera (GI tract).

> Nicotinic receptors are found at the motor end plate, in all autonomic ganglia, and in the adrenal medulla.

Remember the somatic nervous system, which controls movement? It utilizes acetylcholine, and the receptors are all nicotinic. Remember the autonomic ganglia that are present in both the sympathetic and parasympathetic branches? All the preganglionic fibers release acetylcholine, which interacts with nicotinic receptors. Simply make a mental note that the adrenal medulla contains nicotinic receptors and you'll have it made.

Now on to the receptors for NE. Students often find these confusing and difficult to learn.

> Receptors for NE are divided into α and β receptors. These receptors are further subdivided, into α_1 and α_2, and β_1, β_2, and β_3, respectively.

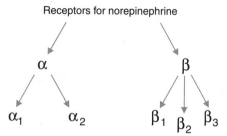

Receptors for norepinephrine

α   β

α₁   α₂   β₁   β₂   β₃

FIGURE 6–6 The subtypes of receptors for NE are illustrated.

There are other α and β receptors, but you should focus here on the five subtypes shown in Figure 6–6. These receptors are found in particular target organs. For example, the heart contains mostly β_1 receptors, while β_2 receptors are found in skeletal muscle blood vessels and the bronchial smooth muscle, and β_3 receptors are found in adipose tissue. This localization of receptor type is the basis of drug therapy. In order to target drug action to the correct organ, drugs have been identified (or designed) that affect only one or two receptor types. This is a very important principle of pharmacology and drug therapy.

GENERAL RULES OF INNERVATION

Many organs are innervated by both the sympathetic and parasympathetic nervous systems. Most of the time the two systems have opposing effects.

When the sympathetic and parasympathetic nervous systems both innervate the same organ system, they tend to have opposite actions. When considering these actions, remember that the sympathetic system (no matter which receptor type is involved) is mediating the fight-or-flight response. For example, both the sympathetic and parasympathetic systems innervate the heart. The sympathetic system increases heart rate and contractility (in order to run faster), while the parasympathetic system decreases heart rate (in order to conserve energy). The one exception to the opposite-effect rule is the salivary glands. Both the sympathetic and parasympathetic systems increase secretion in the salivary glands, but the secretions are of different types.

Important organs that receive innervation from both the sympathetic and parasympathetic nervous systems include the heart, eye, bronchial smooth muscle, GI tract smooth muscle, and genitourinary tract smooth muscle.

In the preceding box, note the absence of the smooth muscles throughout the vascular system (in the arteries).

In the resting state (not in fight-or-flight situations), most dually innervated organs are controlled by the parasympathetic system.

This state dependence is important when considering drug action. At rest, a drug that blocks the effects of NE (sympathetic) will have little effect, whereas a drug that blocks the effects of acetylcholine at muscarinic receptors (parasympathetic) will have a powerful effect. In contrast, in a situation that is dominated by a fight-or-flight response (such as acute trauma or a highly stressful situation), the blocker of NE will have a greater effect.

Most textbooks include a detailed table of target organs listing the effects of activation of the sympathetic versus the parasympathetic nervous system. Look through the table and first rationalize the sympathetic responses to the fight-or-flight response: the pupils should dilate, the heart rate and contractility should increase, the bronchioles should dilate, the GI tract should shut down (the walls relax and the sphincters contract), the bladder should shut down (the walls relax and the sphincter contracts), blood should be shunted from the GI tract and skin to the muscles, and metabolism should increase the supply of glucose. This makes sense and doesn't need to be memorized.

> Most of the vascular smooth muscle is innervated solely by the sympathetic nervous system. This means that blood pressure and peripheral resistance are controlled by the sympathetic nervous system.

Remember that the vascular smooth muscle is the prime example of a target organ that does not have dual innervation.

> Contraction of the radial muscle (sympathetic innervation) causes dilation, or mydriasis (expected sympathetic response), while contraction of the circular muscle (parasympathetic innervation) causes constriction or miosis (expected parasympathetic response).

The responses in the eye can trip up students. One way to remember these responses is to recognize that the ra$d$ial muscle causes $d$ilation (my$d$riasis) and the circular muscle causes constriction (miosis) (that is, there are no d's in any of the words relating to constriction). During your next eye examination, if the doctor dilates your pupils, ask what is in the drops.

> The heart is the main site for β_1 receptors.

If a drug is specific for β_1 receptors, its main effect will be on the heart. β_1 Receptors are also involved in the release of renin from the kidney.

> Activation of β_2 receptors relaxes smooth muscle.

This is somewhat of a generality, but it is useful to help organize your learning. The smooth muscles that contain the β_2 receptors are found in the blood vessels of skeletal muscles (leading to vasodilation), the GI tract, the bronchial walls, the bladder wall, and the pregnant uterus.

> Activation of α receptors causes contraction or constriction, mostly vasoconstriction.

Again, although this statement is a simplification, it is useful to organize your learning. Activation of α receptors contracts blood vessels in the GI tract, contracts the radial muscle in the eye, contracts sphincters in various places, and mediates ejaculation. The latter is the only effect of the sympathetic nervous system that does not fit neatly into fight-or-flight responses.

PRESYNAPTIC RECEPTORS

> Activation of presynaptic α_2 receptors results in feedback inhibition of the release of norepinephrine.

So-called presynaptic receptors are found throughout the central and peripheral nervous systems. The term refers to receptors found on the presynaptic side of the synapse. These receptors are felt to provide feedback to the neuron about the level of activity at the synapse. Activation or inhibition of these receptors can modulate the release of neurotransmitter from the synapse. In the autonomic nervous system, the presynaptic receptor that gets the most attention is the α_2 receptor. Activation of the presynaptic α_2 receptor decreases the release of NE. In essence when a large amount of NE has been released into the synaptic cleft the presynaptic receptors are activated to reduce release of even more NE.

> Inhibition of presynaptic α_2 receptors will increase the release of norepinephrine.

This is where thinking about presynaptic receptors gets tricky. If we inhibit the presynaptic receptor, then the neuron thinks that there is not enough neurotransmitter being released and it increases the release.

7

Cholinergic Agonists

Organization of Class
Direct Cholinergic Agonists
Cholinesterase Inhibitors

ORGANIZATION OF CLASS

Although I have titled this chapter "Cholinergic Agonists," this chapter, in fact, considers all the drugs that increase activity in cholinergic neurons, sometimes called cholinomimetics (because they mimic the action of acetylcholine). There are two main targets of drug action: the postsynaptic receptor and the acetylcholinesterase enzyme, which breaks down acetylcholine.

> Direct-acting cholinergic agonists have a direct action on the receptor for acetylcholine. Some drugs are specific for the muscarinic receptor; others are specific for the nicotinic receptor.

First, remind yourself where the nicotinic and muscarinic receptors are found:

1. *All* autonomic ganglia have nicotinic receptors.
2. *All* receptors at the neuromuscular junction are nicotinic receptors.
3. *All* target organs of the parasympathetic nervous system have muscarinic receptors.

Of course, there are other cholinergic receptors, such as those located in the central nervous system (CNS) and in sweat glands innervated by the sympathetic nervous system. Concentrate on learning the three types listed above for now and add the others later.

> The indirect-acting cholinomimetics act by blocking the metabolism of acetylcholine by cholinesterases. These drugs effectively increase the concentration of acetylcholine at *all* cholinergic synapses.

The enzyme that is specific for acetylcholine is called acetylcholinesterase, and it is found on both the pre- and postsynaptic membranes. There are other cholinesterases that also metabolize acetylcholine and drugs with related structures. These other cholinesterases are sometimes called pseudocholinesterases or nonspecific cholinesterases, and they are abundant in the liver. The structure and biochemistry of acetylcholinesterase is well studied and an interesting story. Details can be found in most textbooks.

Activation of Muscarinic Receptors Results in the Following Responses:

Eye	Miosis (constriction of pupil)
Cardiovascular	Decrease in heart rate
Respiratory	Bronchial constriction and increased secretions
Gastrointestinal (GI)	Increased motility, relaxation of sphincters
Genitourinary (GU)	Relaxation of sphincters and bladder wall contraction
Glands	Increased secretions

Activation of nicotinic receptors results in muscle contraction (fasciculations and weakness).

These effects can be predicted based on your knowledge of the effects of the parasympathetic nervous system. Therefore, this is a review and not a list of new things to learn. (We are trying to keep this simple.)

DIRECT CHOLINERGIC AGONISTS

Esters	Alkaloids
BETHANECHOL	arecoline
carbachol	muscarine
cevimeline	pilocarpine
methacholine	

These drugs are traditionally divided into two groups: esters of choline that are structurally related to acetylcholine (indicated by "-chol-" in their names), and alkaloids that are not related to acetylcholine and are generally plant derivatives. The only reason that this distinction is important is that the alkaloids, because of their complex structure, are not metabolized by cholinesterases.

The effects of *all* of these agents are exclusively muscarinic.

The preceding statement is sweeping and not entirely true. However, the therapeutically useful drugs in reasonable concentrations are muscarinic. The effects of these drugs were listed earlier, but also can be deduced from your knowledge of the parasympathetic nervous system. The differences between the drugs are related to their resistance to cholinesterase activity and specificity for nicotinic receptors.

> BETHANECHOL is used in the treatment of urinary retention.

Of the drugs in this group, bethanechol is the most clinically useful. It is used to treat patients with urinary retention in the postoperative period and in those with a neurogenic bladder.

> The side effects of these drugs are directly related to their interaction with muscarinic receptors.

If you know the actions of these drugs, you also know their side effects. That means there are no new lists to memorize. Side effects often listed for these drugs include sweating (increased secretion), salivation, GI distress, and cramps (due to increased motility).

> Nicotine is a direct agonist at nicotinic receptors.

Nicotine is used therapeutically to help patients stop smoking.

CHOLINESTERASE INHIBITORS

These drugs are often divided into two or three groups based on their structure. Words such as *mono-quaternary amine, bis-quaternary amine, carbamate,* and *organophosphate* appear in many textbooks as names for these subgroups. For our purposes, we'll divide these drugs into two groups: reversible inhibitors, which are water soluble, and irreversible inhibitors (organophosphates), which are lipid soluble.

Reversible Inhibitors		Irreversible Inhibitors
Myasthenia Gravis	**Alzheimer Disease**	
EDROPHONIUM	DONEPEZIL	diisopropyl fluorophosphate
NEOSTIGMINE	galantamine	echothiophate
PYRIDOSTIGMINE	RIVASTIGMINE	isoflurophate
ambenonium	tacrine	malathion
demecarium		parathion
physostigmine		sarin
		soman

The reversible inhibitors include the quaternary amines and the carbamates and are the clinically useful drugs. They compete with acetylcholine for the active site on the cholinesterase enzyme. This group includes the drugs with names ending in "-stigmine" and "-nium."

The irreversible inhibitors phosphorylate the enzyme and inactivate it. These cholinesterase inhibitors are widely used as insecticides and are commonly referred to as nerve gases. Because the organophosphates are lipid soluble, they rapidly cross all membranes, including skin and the blood–brain barrier.

> These drugs have all the same actions (and side effects) as the direct-acting drugs (muscarinic). In addition, because they increase the concentration of acetylcholine, they have effects at the neuromuscular junction (nicotinic).

These drugs will cause the same side effects as the direct cholinergic agonists. There is nothing new here. They also affect nicotinic receptors, primarily at the neuromuscular junction. This is the basis of their therapeutic use. They cause fasciculations and weakness in normal people and can improve muscle strength in patients with myasthenia gravis. Myasthenia gravis is an immune disease in which there is loss of acetylcholine receptors at the neuromuscular junction, resulting in weakness and fatigability of skeletal muscle.

These drugs can have effects on the cholinergic system in the CNS, if the drug can cross the blood–brain barrier. The effects range from tremor, anxiety, and restlessness to coma. The organophosphates, because of their lipid solubility, rapidly cross into the CNS.

> EDROPHONIUM is used in the diagnosis of myasthenia gravis.

Edrophonium is a short-acting cholinesterase inhibitor that is administered intravenously to patients suspected of having weakness caused by myasthenia gravis. If they have myasthenia gravis, the drug will dramatically improve muscle strength. If they do not have myasthenia gravis, what do you think the effects of administration of a cholinesterase inhibitor would be?*

> NEOSTIGMINE, PYRIDOSTIGMINE, and ambenonium are used in the treatment of myasthenia gravis.

These three drugs act in the same way as edrophonium, but are longer acting. Therefore, they are used for treatment and not for diagnosis.

> Other uses of the reversible cholinesterase inhibitors: treatment of open-angle glaucoma, treatment of Alzheimer disease and the reversal of nondepolarizing neuromuscular blockade after surgery.

---

*These effects could include increased secretions and GI cramping (because of increased motility).

Studies have shown a deficiency of cholinergic neurons in patients with Alzheimer disease. There are currently four acetylcholinesterase drugs available to delay symptomatic progression of the disease, although tacrine is rarely used. None of these agents reverse the disease or ultimately prevent progression. These drugs are able to work because they have more efficacy in the brain than peripherally. Other drugs in this class can be used in open-angle glaucoma and for reversal of nondepolarizing neuromuscular blockade after surgery.

> There are no therapeutic uses for the irreversible cholinesterase inhibitors.

These agents are of interest because of the biochemistry involved in the drug-enzyme interaction and because poisoning with these agents is common. In 1995, sarin gas was released by a terrorist cult group into three different subway lines in Tokyo injuring more than 5500 people.

> PRALIDOXIME and ATROPINE are used to treat poisoning with organophosphates.

The organophosphates phosphorylate the cholinesterase enzyme, thus inactivating it. Pralidoxime is able to hydrolyze the phosphate bond and reactivate the enzyme. This works well if the enzyme-phosphate complex has not "aged" (a story too complex to be included in this book, but quite interesting). In addition, because pralidoxime does not cross the blood–brain barrier, it is not effective in reversing the CNS effects of the organophosphates. Atropine (a muscarinic antagonist) is used in organophosphate poisoning because it will block the effects of the excess acetylcholine, but only at the muscarinic receptors. It has no effect at the neuromuscular junction (nicotinic).

Cholinergic Antagonists

8

- Organization of Class
- Muscarinic Antagonists
- Ganglionic Blockers
- Neuromuscular Blockers

ORGANIZATION OF CLASS

The drugs in this group antagonize the effects of acetylcholine. Most of these drugs are antagonists directly at the nicotinic or muscarinic receptor. Some act on the ion channel associated with the nicotinic receptor, and still others block acetylcholine release.

MUSCARINIC ANTAGONISTS

> The prototypic muscarinic antagonist is ATROPINE.

In this group of compounds it is useful to consider a prototype drug and then compare the other drugs to it. The prototype drug for the muscarinic antagonists is atropine.

> All of the muscarinic antagonists are competitive antagonists for the binding of acetylcholine to the muscarinic receptor.

These drugs compete with acetylcholine for binding to the muscarinic receptor. They have no intrinsic activity. In other words, in the absence of acetylcholine, they would have no effect.

The effects and side effects of these drugs are the opposite of the drugs considered in the previous chapter (the cholinomimetics)

Eye	Mydriasis, cycloplegia (blurred vision)
Skin	Reduced sweating, flushing
Gastrointestinal (GI)	Reduced motility and secretions
Cardiovascular	Increased heart rate (high doses)
Respiratory	Bronchial dilation and decreased secretion
Genitourinary (GU)	Urinary retention
Central nervous system (CNS)	Drowsiness, hallucinations, coma

Compare these effects to those listed in the corresponding box in Chapter 7. The important ones to remember are the common side effects of drugs that have anticholinergic properties (many of the CNS drugs); that is, dry eyes, dry mouth, blurred vision, constipation, and urinary retention. If you master the anticholinergic effects now, it will save you considerable effort later.

Many muscarinic antagonists are currently available and their names do not all sound alike. Some name recognition exercises may be useful here.

Muscarinic Antagonists

ATROPINE	benztropine	pirenzepine
IPRATROPIUM	cyclopentolate	propantheline
SCOPOLAMINE	darifenacin	solifenacin
	dicyclomine	tolterodine
	fesoterodine	trihexyphenidyl
	glycopyrrolate	tropicamide
	oxybutinin	trospium
	oxybutynin	

Some of these drugs have particular uses. Learn the names of these drugs first and add the others later.

Muscarinic antagonists are used preoperatively to reduce secretions.

SCOPOLAMINE is used to prevent motion sickness.

Scopolamine has an effect in the CNS to reduce motion sickness. It is usually administered using a transdermal patch.

> IPRATROPIUM is used in the treatment of chronic obstructive pulmonary disease (COPD) to produce bronchodilation.

As you know from Chapter 6, activation of β_2 receptors will result in relaxation of the smooth muscle in the bronchial tree. Thus, β_2 agonists will produce bronchodilation. So will muscarinic antagonists, such as ipratropium and tiotropium. Whether to use a β_2 agonist or a muscarinic antagonist in a particular patient has to do with the underlying pathophysiology of the pulmonary disease and the side-effect profiles of the different bronchodilators.

> Muscarinic antagonists are used for urinary frequency, urgency, and urge incontinence caused by bladder (detrusor) overactivity.

Detrusor overactivity is a common cause of urinary incontinence in elderly patients. As you might expect, these drugs cause dry mouth and constipation.

Other drugs in this group are used to produce mydriasis and to treat patients with Parkinson disease, and as adjuncts in the treatment of irritable bowel syndrome.

GANGLIONIC BLOCKERS

Ganglionic blockers work by interfering with the postsynaptic action of acetylcholine. They block the action of acetylcholine at the nicotinic receptor of all autonomic ganglia. These drugs are very rarely used clinically.

NEUROMUSCULAR BLOCKERS

These drugs are a little out of place in a section on drugs affecting the autonomic nervous system. However, because they block the effects of acetylcholine by interacting with nicotinic receptors, we'll consider them here. Inclusion here also makes it easier to learn about these drugs and their side effects.

> The competitive neuromuscular blocking drugs are used to produce skeletal muscle relaxation.

All of these drugs bind to all nicotinic receptors (at the neuromuscular junction and autonomic ganglia) and some actually bind muscarinic receptors to a small extent. The neuromuscular blockers act relatively selectively at the nicotinic receptor at the neuromuscular junction. They vary in their potency and in their duration of action.

The drugs are classified as depolarizing or nondepolarizing blockers based on their mechanism of action. The depolarizing blocker binds to the receptor and opens the ion channel, resulting in depolarization of the end plate (hence its name). The nondepolarizing blockers bind to the receptor, but do not open the ion channel.

The effects of all of these drugs can be reversed by administration of a cholinesterase inhibitor (to increase the amount of acetylcholine available to compete with the receptor blocker). A muscarinic antagonist is often administered at the same time. Can you rationalize why? Hint: You only want to increase the acetylcholine concentration at the neuromuscular junction, which is nicotinic, but the cholinesterase inhibitor works everywhere.

> SUCCINYLCHOLINE is a depolarizing neuromuscular blocker.

To make things simpler, there is only one depolarizing agent that you need to know: succinylcholine. Succinylcholine will depolarize the neuromuscular junction. It has a brief action, and its use has been associated with malignant hyperthermia, which can be *fatal*.

Now, let's move on to the nondepolarizing blockers. There are several of these.

Nondepolarizing Blockers

d-TUBOCURARINE	mivacurium
atracurium	PANCURONIUM
cisatracurium	pipecuronium
doxacurium	rocuronium
gallamine	vecuronium
metocurine iodide	

Notice that most of the drug names contain the letters "-cur-". This should make it easier to recognize the drugs in this group when you see them.

The neuromuscular junction (and other cholinergic synapses) can also be blocked by drugs that block the release of acetylcholine.

> Botulinum toxin blocks the release of acetylcholine at all cholinergic synapses.

We usually think of botulinum toxin as a very potent poison that causes botulism. However, it has found a therapeutic use in the treatment of prolonged muscle spasm and for excessive sweating. A small amount of the toxin is injected directly into a muscle fiber paralyzing the muscle, or in the skin blocking stimulation of the sweat glands. Botulinum toxin is also being used to "treat" wrinkles.

> DANTROLENE is used to treat malignant hyperthermia.

That was a short aside. There was no good place to put dantrolene, and you need to know its name and use. You may also wish to learn its mechanism of action. It interfers with release of calcium from the sarcoplasmic reticulum in skeletal muscle.

Adrenergic Agonists

Organization of Class
Direct-Acting Agonists
Dopamine
Indirect-Acting Agents
Cardiovascular Effects of Norepinephrine, Epinephrine, and Isoproterenol

ORGANIZATION OF CLASS

This chapter considers the drugs that mimic the effects of adrenergic nerve stimulation (or stimulation of the adrenal medulla). In other words, these compounds mimic the effects of norepinephrine or epinephrine. These drugs are sometimes referred to as adrenomimetics or sympathomimetics. Remember that the actions of the sympathetic nervous system are mediated through α and β receptors.

Remember that:

α_1 = most vascular smooth muscle; agonists contract

β_1 = heart; agonists increase rate

β_2 = respiratory and uterine smooth muscle; agonists relax

There are other effects of sympathetic stimulation, but the three listed in the preceding box are the most important.

Suppose you have as a patient a 65-year-old man with a long history of reactive airway disease. He recently had a mild heart attack. Now he has come to you because of a flare-up of his airway disease. You want to relax the smooth muscle of the bronchials without stimulating the heart (you don't want to jeopardize his heart function by increasing the cardiac workload). If you could stimulate the β_2 receptors in the respiratory tract specifically, then you could successfully treat this patient. This example illustrates why it is important to know where the receptors are located and which drugs are specific for which receptors.

The adrenergic agonists are often divided into direct- and indirect-acting agonists. This is a useful distinction for a number of reasons. The indirect-acting drugs do not bind to specific receptors, but act by releasing stored norepinephrine. This means that their actions are nonspecific. The direct-acting drugs bind to the receptors, so specificity of action is a possibility.

The drugs are also sometimes divided into catecholamines and noncatecholamines. This is yet another division based on structure (and our focus here is not on structures). However, this distinction is useful for one concept. Do you remember from Chapter 6 that norepinephrine is metabolized by catechol-o-methyltransferase (COMT) and monoamine oxidase (MAO)? Well, the other catecholamines are also metabolized by these enzymes; however, the noncatecholamines are not.

DIRECT-ACTING AGONISTS

The focus here is to learn the specificity of the drugs for their receptor targets. If you know the effect of stimulation of the target receptors, then you can deduce the drug actions and adverse effects.

> Only EPINEPHRINE and NOREPINEPHRINE activate both α and β receptors.

Although this is an oversimplification, it provides a useful starting point. The rest of the direct-acting drugs act on *either* α or β receptors (Figure 9–1). Epinephrine has approximately equal effects at α and β receptors. In addition, it has approximately equal effects at β_1 and β_2 receptors.

Epinephrine has a number of uses, including the treatment of allergic reactions and shock, the control of localized bleeding, and the prolongation of the action of local anesthetics.

> NOREPINEPHRINE has a relatively low affinity for β_2 receptors.

Norepinephrine activates both α and β receptors, but activates β_1 receptors more than β_2 receptors. Because of its relatively low affinity for β_2 receptors, norepinephrine is not as useful in the treatment of bronchospasm as epinephrine. Why? Because the smooth muscle of the bronchioles are relaxed by activation of β_2 receptors.

Now let's move on to consider the α- and β-specific drugs. The α-specific drugs are easier, so let's begin there.

Drug	Receptor Effect	Clinical Effect
PHENYLEPHRINE	α_1 agonist	Nasal decongestant
CLONIDINE	α_2 agonist	Decreases blood pressure through a central action

The main effect of α_1 stimulation (with an agonist such as phenylephrine) is vasoconstriction. Local application of a vasoconstrictor to the nasal passages decreases blood flow locally and decreases secretions, thus acting as a nasal decongestant. The action of clonidine is more complex. It activates α_2 receptors in the central nervous system to decrease sympathetic stimulation to the heart and activates presynaptic α_2 receptors on peripheral nerve endings to inhibit the release of norepinephrine.

Drug	Receptor Effect	Clinical Effect
DOBUTAMINE	β_1 agonist	Increases heart rate and cardiac output
ISOPROTERENOL	$\beta_1 = \beta_2$ agonist	
ALBUTEROL	β_2 agonist	Relieve bronchoconstriction
TERBUTALINE		
metaproterenol		

Basically, the affinity of these drugs for receptors falls on a spectrum from β_1 to β_2 (see Figure 9–1). Dobutamine is closer to the β_1 end of the spectrum; terbutaline and its relatives are closer to the β_2 end. Isoproterenol falls in the middle of the spectrum. The action of dobutamine is actually quite complex and worth reading about.

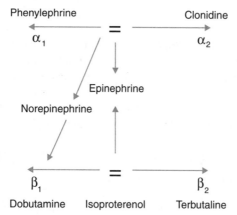

FIGURE 9–1 A classification of adrenergic agonists is presented. Affinity for the α receptors is shown at the top of the diagram and affinity for the β receptors at the bottom. Epinephrine and norepinephrine have affinity for both α and β receptors and are, therefore, placed in the middle.

DOPAMINE

Dopamine is a catecholamine by structure and is a precursor to norepinephrine (see Figure 6–3). Dopamine receptors are located throughout the body and in the central nervous system. At high doses dopamine acts much like epinephrine.

At low doses, DOPAMINE causes renal and coronary vasodilation. It also activates β_1 receptors in the heart.

In the treatment of shock, dopamine increases heart rate and cardiac output while simultaneously dilating the renal and coronary arteries. The action of dopamine in the renal vascular bed is useful in attempts to preserve renal blood flow and renal function in the presence of overall decreased tissue perfusion (shock).

INDIRECT-ACTING AGENTS

> The indirect-acting sympathomimetic agents act by releasing previously stored norepinephrine.

Because these drugs act by releasing stored norepinephrine, their effects are widespread and nonspecific. Ephedrine and phenylpropanolamine are nasal decongestants. Phenylpropanolamine has also been used as an appetite suppressant. Don't worry if you can't remember these drugs. Be careful, however, not to confuse phenylephrine (the specific α_1 agonist) with these two similarly named indirect agents.

> AMPHETAMINE and its relatives, dexmethylphenidate and methylphenidate, are central nervous system stimulants used to treat attention deficit hyperactivity disorder in children.

Amphetamine and its other relatives are indirect-acting sympathomimetics that have been abused because of their psychostimulant abilities. There are quite a number of formulations of amphetamine producing differing durations of action and abuse potential. The somnolence of narcoplepsy has treated with methylphenidate, but newer drugs, modafinil and armodafinil are now available and have less abuse potential. The mechanism of action of modafinil is not understood.

CARDIOVASCULAR EFFECTS OF NOREPINEPHRINE, EPINEPHRINE, AND ISOPROTERENOL

Before we leave the adrenergic activators, it is useful to consider in detail the cardiovascular actions of epinephrine, norepinephrine, and isoproterenol. Some textbooks will also consider dopamine in this context. Consider the effects of these agents on heart rate, cardiac output, total peripheral resistance, and mean arterial pressure. If you find these effects easy enough to remember, try adding their effects on systolic and diastolic blood pressure to your mental database.

> Norepinephrine increases total peripheral resistance and mean arterial pressure.

Through stimulation of α receptors, norepinephrine causes constriction of all major vascular beds. This, in turn, causes an increase in resistance and pressure. The increase in blood pressure causes a reflex increase in parasympathetic output to the heart, which acts to slow the heart down. Therefore, heart rate often decreases after administration of norepinephrine in spite of direct activation of β_1 receptors.

> Epinephrine predominantly affects the heart through β_1 receptors, causing an increase in heart rate and cardiac output.

Although epinephrine activates all α and β receptors, if given systemically its effects are predominated by effects on the heart. It increases heart rate, stroke volume, and cardiac output. The effects of epinephrine on blood pressure and peripheral resistance are dose dependent. At low doses, there is a fall in peripheral resistance as a result of vasodilation in the skeletal muscle beds (β_2 effect). At higher doses, there is some vasoconstriction (α_1) balancing the vasodilation (β_2), resulting in little or no change in peripheral resistance. At even higher doses, the vasoconstriction (α_1) will predominate, resulting in an increase in peripheral resistance and blood pressure.

> Isoproterenol causes a marked decrease in total peripheral resistance and an increase in heart rate and cardiac output.

Remember that isoproterenol is an agonist at all β receptors. Therefore, it does not cause vasoconstriction of the vascular smooth muscle (α_1). The vasodilation in the skeletal muscle beds (β_2) is unopposed. This results in a net decrease in peripheral resistance. Isoproterenol also stimulates β_1 receptors in the heart, resulting in an increase in heart rate and stroke volume.

Which of the graphs in Figure 9–2 represents the changes resulting from administration of epinephrine? Norepinephrine? Isoproterenol?*

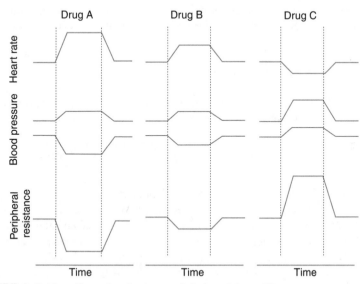

FIGURE 9–2 The effects of an intravenous infusion of three different agents on heart rate, blood pressure (systolic and diastolic), and peripheral vascular resistance are graphed. The drugs were administered during the time indicated by the vertical dashed lines. Which graph represents the effects of epinephrine? Norepinephrine? Isoproterenol?

*Answers: (Drug A) isoproterenol; (Drug B) epinephrine; (Drug C) norepinephrine.

10 Adrenergic Antagonists

Organization of Class
Central Blockers
α-Blockers
β-Blockers
Mixed α- and β-Blockers

ORGANIZATION OF CLASS

The effects of the sympathetic nervous system can be blocked either by decreasing sympathetic outflow from the brain, suppressing release of norepinephrine from terminals, or by blocking postsynaptic receptors. Adrenergic antagonists reduce the effectiveness of sympathetic nerve stimulation and the effects of exogenously applied agonists, such as isoproterenol. Most often the receptor antagonists are divided into α-receptor antagonists and β-receptor antagonists. This classification will work for us also.

CENTRAL BLOCKERS

At this point we are finally ready for a short discussion of α_2-receptor agonists. Yes, I did write agonists, not antagonists—and in a chapter on antagonists.

> α_2 Agonists reduce sympathetic nerve activity and are used to treat hypertension.

α_2-Receptor activation inhibits both sympathetic output from the brain and release of norepinephrine from nerve terminals. We have already listed one of these drugs—clonidine. There are at least two others: guanabenz and guanfacine. α-Methyl-dopa is metabolized to α-methylnorepinephrine, which is also an α_2 agonist. Because the α_2 agonists reduce the output from the brain to the sympathetic nervous system, they have found a use in the treatment of hypertension. Yet another central α_2 agonist, tizanidine, has found use in the treatment of spasticity.

α -BLOCKERS

Many compounds possess some α-blocking activity in addition to their primary action. For example, the antipsychotics have α-antagonist properties. In the case of

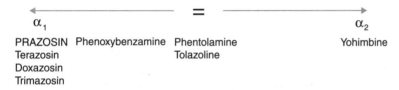

FIGURE 10–1 The relative affinities of various antagonists for the α receptor are schematized.

the antipsychotics, these actions are considered side effects. The drugs that we will consider here have their primary action as α antagonists.

> Most of the α antagonists allow vasodilation and, thus, decrease blood pressure.

Remember that α-receptor activation results in vasoconstriction. It should follow that α-receptor blockade will produce vasodilation. This is particularly true when the sympathetic nervous system is firing. For example, the sympathetic nervous system is more active in maintaining blood pressure when a person is standing than when lying down. This is why α-blockade results in a greater decrease in blood pressure in the standing position. This effect is called postural hypotension.

> The side effects of the α-blockers are directly related to their α-blocking activity.

For the most part, the side effects of the α-blockers are intuitive. The most common of these effects are postural hypotension and reflex tachycardia.

In Chapter 9, we briefly reviewed the subtypes of the α receptors. You could probably have guessed that there are drugs that are specific antagonists for the α_1 receptor and others that are specific for the α_2 receptor (Figure 10–1). As shown in the figure, phentolamine and tolazoline are about equal in effectiveness at the α_1 and α_2 receptors, whereas phenoxybenzamine is a much more effective α_1- than α_2-blocker. The rest of the drugs listed in the figure are selective for the α_1 receptor. Notice that the names in this latter group all end in "-azosin."

> TAMSULOSIN and silodosin are specific antagonists of the α_{1A} receptor and are used in the symptomatic treatment of benign prostatic hypertrophy

Because α_1 receptors mediate contraction in the genitourinary system, α_1 antagonists, such as alfuzosin, can cause the smooth muscle in the bladder neck and prostate to relax and improve urine flow in patients with benign prostatic hypertrophy. Evidence suggests that the subtype of α_1 receptor present in the genitourinary tract is the α_{1A} receptor. Antagonism of this specific receptor reduces the cardiovascular side effects, particularly the orthostatic hypotension.

> All of the α-blockers are reversible inhibitors of the α receptor, except phenoxybenzamine, which is irreversible.

> The "-azosins," such as PRAZOSIN, are used in the treatment of hypertension.

Because of their specificity for α_1 receptors, prazosin and its relatives (terazosin, doxazosin, and trimazosin) have fewer side effects.

Yohimbine is a selective antagonist at α_2 receptors. It has no clinical role.

β-BLOCKERS

To begin, remind yourself of the localization and action of the β receptors. β_1 Receptors are found in the heart, and their activation leads to an increase in heart rate and contractility. β_2 Receptors are found in smooth muscle of the respiratory tract, the uterus, and blood vessels. Their activation leads to relaxation of the smooth muscle.

> Remember that:
>
> β_1 = heart; antagonists decrease rate
>
> β_2 = smooth muscle; antagonists contract
>
> This latter effect translates into bronchial constriction, which may be dangerous in asthmatics.

The actions of β-blockers on blood pressure are complex. Remember that α receptors control most of the vascular smooth muscle in an unopposed fashion. Chronic administration of β-blockers will, however, decrease blood pressure in people with high blood pressure. The mechanism is not fully understood.

> The β-blockers have widespread use in the management of cardiac arrhythmias, angina, and hypertension.

β-Blockers are also used in the treatment of hyperthyroidism, glaucoma, migraines, and anxiety.

> β-Blockers should be used with caution in diabetics.

Recall that the metabolic effects of sympathetic stimulation (glycogenolysis, gluconeogenesis, lipolysis) are mediated by β receptors. In response to hypoglycemia (low blood glucose) the sympathetic nervous system stimulates an increase in blood glucose through β receptors. Blocking this response with a β-blocker will cause the blood glucose to remain low. In addition, the reflex increase in heart rate that occurs in response to hypoglycemia is also blocked by β-blockers. Many diabetics can detect a drop in blood glucose by the reflex increase in heart rate. If you are giving them β-blockers, they lose this early warning sign.

> β_1 Selective antagonists are often referred to as cardioselective.

Most of the β receptors in the heart are β_1 receptors. For this reason, drugs that are selective for the β_1 receptor are referred to as cardioselective.

Nonselective	Beta$_1$-Selective
PROPRANOLOL	acebutolol
carteolol	atenolol
levobunolol	betaxolol
nadolol	bisoprolol
penbutolol	esmolol
pindolol	metoprolol
timolol	

Looking at the names only, there is no good way to distinguish the cardioselective drugs from the others, and it is not really important at this stage to know which they are. On the bright side, every student can recognize the "-olol" ending in the names of the β-blockers.

Besides their receptor selectivity, these drugs vary in duration of action and metabolism.

> The adverse effects of these drugs are, for the most part, directly related to their β-blocking abilities.

The β-blockers can cause bronchoconstriction, decreased heart rate, and cardiac output. Any of these actions could be considered side effects.

> Some β-blockers are said to have intrinsic sympathomimetic activity. This means they have partial agonist activity, even though they are classified as β-blockers.

Students often find the idea of intrinsic sympathomimetic activity confusing. These drugs bind well to the β receptor. In the absence of lots of competing catecholamines, they activate the receptor a little bit. When there are lots of catecholamines, however, these drugs block the receptor from further activation by the catecholamines. Thus, it may be best to simply think of them as partial agonists with high affinity for the receptor. However, they are classified under β-blockers. At this point, it is important to know that some β-blockers have intrinsic sympathomimetic activity but not necessary to memorize the names.

MIXED α- AND β-BLOCKERS

Several drugs are classified as both α- and β-blockers. The oldest of these is labetalol.

First, notice that labetalol does not end in "-olol," but in "-alol." Use this clue to remember that labetalol is different from the other β-blockers.

> Labetalol has both α- and β-blocking activity.

Because of the ratio of β-to-α activity, labetalol is most often listed as a β-blocker with some α-blocking activity. It is nonselective at the β receptor, but is specific for α_1 receptors. Its effects are rather complex, but make for interesting reading. You can use the mechanism of action of this drug to test your understanding of the adrenergic receptors and their actions.

A newer mixed antagonist is carvedilol. It is listed as a nonselective β blocker with no intrinsic sympathomimetic activity and as an α_1-blocker. This makes it very similar to labetalol. As with labetalol, notice how its spelling (the "-ilol" ending) provides a clue to the different action of this drug.

PART III Drugs That Affect the Cardiovascular System

CHAPTER 11: Antihypertensive Drugs   59

CHAPTER 12: Drugs Used in Ischemic Heart
             Disease and Congestive Heart Failure   69

CHAPTER 13: Antiarrhythmic Drugs   73

CHAPTER 14: Drugs That Affect Blood   79

CHAPTER 15: Lipid-Lowering Drugs   86

Antihypertensive Drugs

Organization of Class
Diuretics
Drugs That Interfere with the Renin-Angiotensin System
    Angiotensin-Converting Enzyme (ACE) Inhibitors
    Angiotensin II Receptor Blockers (ARBs)
    Selective Aldosterone Receptor Antagonists
Direct Renin Inhibitor (DRI)
Calcium Channel Blockers
Nitrates
Other Direct Vasodilators
α- and β-Blockers
Clonidine

ORGANIZATION OF CLASS

High blood pressure (hypertension) develops when the blood volume is large compared to the available space in the blood vessels. The control of blood pressure is complex and involves vascular, cardiac, and renal physiology.

Mean arterial pressure = Cardiac output × Peripheral resistance

The preceding equation should be familiar from physiology. According to this equation, a decrease in either cardiac output or peripheral resistance will decrease blood pressure. Conversely, if high blood pressure is present, something must have increased one of the two variables.

A number of factors will increase cardiac output, including increased heart rate, increased contractility, and increased sodium and water retention. Vasoconstriction will increase peripheral resistance. Decreasing one or more of these factors is the goal of antihypertensive therapy.

Diuretics can be used to decrease blood volume. Drugs are available that interfere with the renin-angiotensin system, which is intimately involved in salt and water balance in the body. Finally, drugs can be used to decrease peripheral vascular resistance or cardiac output. This can be done with direct-acting vasodilators or by using agents that block sympathetic nervous system output.

I. Diuretics
   A. Thiazides
   B. Loop diuretics
   C. Potassium (K⁺)-sparing diuretics
II. Drugs that interfere with the renin-angiotensin system
   A. ACE inhibitors
   B. Angiotensin II receptor antagonists (ARBs)
   C. Aldosterone antagonists
   D. Direct renin inhibitor (DRI)
III. Drugs that decrease peripheral vascular resistance or cardiac output
   A. Direct vasodilators
      1. Calcium channel blockers
      2. Nitrates
   B. Sympathetic nervous system depressants
      1. α- and β-Blockers
      2. Clonidine

As you can see from this outline, it is easiest to organize the antihypertensive drugs by their mechanism of action. Some of these drugs are also useful in the treatment of angina or heart failure.

DIURETICS

Drugs that increase urine flow are called diuretics. Diuretics play an important role in the management of high blood pressure. They are often used in combination with other classes of antihypertensive drugs. These drugs are ion transport inhibitors in the kidney, so a short review of renal physiology may be useful for you at this point.

There are basically three groups of diuretics, named according to their structure and mechanism of action: thiazide diuretics, loop diuretics, and potassium-sparing diuretics. Consider the group names for these drugs; in particular, the phrase *potassium sparing*. This should tell you that the other two groups cause a *loss* of potassium. You now know a major side effect of both the thiazide diuretics and the loop diuretics. Next consider the name *loop* diuretics. If you had to guess the site of action of these drugs, what would you guess? I am sure you said the loop of Henle. So you see, you already know the site of action of this group.

Thiazide Diuretics	Loop Diuretics	Potassium-Sparing Diuretics
CHLOROTHIAZIDE	FUROSEMIDE	SPIRONOLACTONE
HYDROCHLOROTHIAZIDE	bumetanide	amiloride
chlorthalidone	ethacrynic acid	triamterene
metolazone	torsemide	eplerenone
indapamide		
hydroflumethiazide		

Name recognition is extremely important with these drugs. Many a student has missed an exam (or board) question because he or she didn't recognize a drug as a potassium-sparing diuretic. This recognition is made more difficult by the fact that the names of these drugs do not have similar endings (or beginnings).

> The thiazide diuretics inhibit sodium and chloride reabsorption in the thick ascending loop of Henle and early distal tubule (Figure 11–1). This loss of ions increases urine volume.

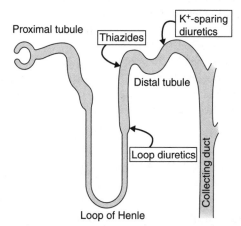

FIGURE 11–1 The location of action of the different classes of diuretics is illustrated here. The loop diuretics act in the ascending loop of Henle. The thiazide diuretics and potassium (K)-sparing diuretics act in the distal tubule.

> The thiazide diuretics are the *drugs of choice* in the treatment of primary hypertension.

Primary hypertension is high blood pressure for which no cause can be found. Thiazide diuretics have been shown to decrease mortality in patients with hypertension. The diuretic effect of thiazides is not solely responsible for their effectiveness as antihypertensives (Figure 11–2).

> The thiazide diuretics can cause hypokalemia.

But you already know this, don't you? If not, simply remember that thiazides are *not* potassium-sparing diuretics.

> The loop diuretics inhibit chloride reabsorption in the thick ascending loop of Henle.

Their action in the loop of Henle gives the loop diuretics their name. Now you simply need to remember that these drugs inhibit chloride reabsorption.

> The loop diuretics are commonly used to reduce pulmonary edema in patients with congestive heart failure.

Loop diuretics are used in the treatment of pulmonary edema because of their potency and rapid onset of action. Loop diuretics are also useful in treating patients with hypertension caused by renal insufficiency.

> The major side effect of the loop diuretics is hypokalemia.

Again, there is nothing new in this statement. The loop diuretics are more potent than the thiazide diuretics. They are the preferred diuretics in patients with low glomerular filtration rates. They can cause a host of metabolic abnormalities, the most common being hypokalemia (low K^+). Dehydration can also be a problem. Finally, they can increase the toxicity of drugs that cause damage to the ear (ototoxicity) and to the kidney (nephrotoxicity).

The potassium-sparing diuretics enhance sodium excretion and retain potassium by an action in the distal tubule. The potassium-sparing diuretics are often used in combination with the other diuretics to help maintain the potassium balance. They can cause hyperkalemia. Alone, the potassium-sparing diuretics are not very potent.

DRUGS THAT INTERFERE WITH THE RENIN-ANGIOTENSIN SYSTEM

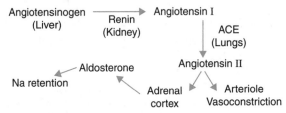

FIGURE 11–2 The renin-angiotensin-aldosterone system.

The renin-angiotensin system plays a central role in the regulation of fluid balance in the body. Before moving on to the drugs that interfere in this system, take a few moments to review the physiology (Figure 11–2).

ANGIOTENSIN-CONVERTING ENZYME (ACE) INHIBITORS

Angiotensin-converting enzyme (ACE, also known as peptidyldipeptide hydrolase or peptidyl dipeptidase) converts angiotensin I to angiotensin II, which is a potent vasoconstrictor and stimulator of aldosterone secretion. Aldosterone promotes sodium and water retention and potassium excretion. This leads to an increase in vascular volume and an increase in peripheral vascular resistance.

> ACE inhibitors block the synthesis of angiotensin II.

Blocking the synthesis of angiotensin II leads to a decrease in levels of this circulating vasoconstrictor, which results in a decrease in blood pressure (that is, afterload). ACE inhibitors also reduce aldosterone secretion, which results in a net water loss. This adds to the decrease in afterload.

The currently available ACE inhibitors prils are listed in the following table. Feel free to add to this list as needed.

ACE Inhibitors

CAPTOPRIL	moexipril
ENALAPRIL	perindopril
benazepril	quinapril
fosinopril	ramipril
lisinopril	trandolapril

ACE inhibitors have several uses, most prominently in the treatment of patients with hypertension and heart failure (see Chapter 12). In hypertensive patients, ACE inhibitors reduce blood pressure while causing little or no change in cardiac output. The antihypertensive effects of the ACE inhibitors are additive with the effects of many other drugs.

These drugs are particularly useful in hypertension that is a result of increased renin levels. Because they do not affect glucose levels, ACE inhibitors are also used in the treatment of diabetic patients with hypertension. ACE inhibitors have been shown to preserve renal function in patients with nephropathy. The major side effects of these drugs are headache, dizziness, abdominal pain, confusion, renal failure, and impotence. ACE inhibitors can also cause a cough.

ANGIOTENSIN II RECEPTOR BLOCKERS (ARBS)

Angiotensin II Receptor blockers

candesartan
eprosartan
losartan
irbesartan
olmesartan
telmisartan
valsartan

Notice that, so far, the names of the drugs in the preceding box all end in "-sartan." However, this is no guarantee that new ones under development will retain the "-sartan" ending.

> The ARBs interfere with the binding of angiotensin II with its receptor.

These drugs prevent activation of the angiotensin receptor; hence, their actions are very similar to the actions of ACE inhibitors, which block the formation of angiotensin II. ARBs are as effective in lowering blood pressure and also just as cardio- and renal protective as the ACE inhibitors with fewer side effects.

SELECTIVE ALDOSTERONE RECEPTOR ANTAGONISTS

> Spironolactone and eplerenone are antagonists of aldosterone at the mineralocorticoid receptor and can be used to treat hypertension.

Remember that aldosterone promotes sodium and water retention and potassium excretion which leads to an increase in vascular volume and vascular resistance. Blocking the action of the aldosterone receptor will increase urinary excretion of sodium.

DIRECT RENIN INHIBITOR (DRI)

Aliskiren is the first direct renin inhibitor available. It binds in the pocket of the renin enzyme that is essential for its activity. Whether aliskiren offers any advantages over the ACE inhibitors or ARBs remains to be determined.

CALCIUM CHANNEL BLOCKERS

Calcium Channel Blockers

DILTIAZEM	amlodipine
NIFEDIPINE	felodipine
VERAPAMIL	isradipine
	nicardipine
	nisoldipine
	clevidipine

There are many calcium channel blockers, and the list seems to grow longer every year. These agents differ in pharmacokinetic properties, potency, and selectivity of action. The names of the calcium channel blockers all end in "-di-pine," "-mil," or "-dil," except diltiazem. Don't confuse diltiazem with diazepam (a benzodiazepine that is used as a sedative; see Chapter 17).

> Calcium channel blockers inhibit the entry of calcium into cells. They cause a decrease in afterload.

If the preceding statements sounded simplistic, they were meant to. This is another instance where the mechanism of action gives a group of drugs its name.

Vascular tone and contraction are largely determined by the availability of extracellular calcium. When the entry of calcium into smooth muscle cells of the arteries is inhibited, the vessels will dilate. The cardiac response to the decrease in vascular resistance is variable.

> The most common side effects of the calcium channel blockers (headaches, dizziness, hypotension, etc.) are related to vasodilation.

Remember that the side effects of these drugs are a direct extension of their action. This means you have nothing new to memorize.

NITRATES

Nitrates

NITROGLYCERIN
amyl nitrite
isosorbide dinitrate
isosorbide mononitrate

Notice that the drugs in this class all have "nitro-," "-nitrate," or "nitrite" in their names. This makes them easy to identify. The nitrates reduce blood pressure, but, except for some special instances, they are not commonly used in the treatment of patients with hypertension. As vasodilators, however, they fit into this chapter.

> The nitrates dilate blood vessels and reduce cardiac preload.

Although these drugs have been in use for many years, their mechanism of action is not completely clear (in fact, it is actually rather muddy). It is now thought that these drugs work by conversion to nitric oxide. The nitric oxide increases intracellular cGMP, which leads to smooth muscle relaxation. At higher concentrations the nitrates decrease afterload.

> NITROGLYCERIN is the most commonly used antianginal agent. It is the *drug of choice* for relieving acute coronary spasm.

Nitroglycerin is often administered sublingually for rapid onset of action, but it can be applied transdermally for a longer duration of action. If taken orally, it is subject to extensive first-pass metabolism in the liver. Its effectiveness against coronary spasm suggests a direct vasodilatory effect on the coronary arteries.

Isosorbide dinitrate is an orally active nitrate that has a relatively long half-life.

> NITROPRUSSIDE is a vasodilator given by continuous IV infusion. It is rapidly metabolized to cyanide.

Nitroprusside is used in hypertensive emergencies to rapidly bring down a dangerously high blood pressure. The blood pressure can be controlled with small changes in the IV infusion rate.

> Headaches and postural hypotension are common side effects of the use of nitrates.

These side effects do not need to be memorized. It is easy to see that they are directly related to the mechanism of action of the nitrates (vasodilation). Too much vasodilation peripherally leads to postural hypotension (the blood vessels cannot contract and maintain blood pressure when a person stands up), and dilation of cerebral vessels is thought to lead to headaches.

There is also the interesting problem of patient tolerance to the effects of nitrates. It is too low down on the trivia list to include here. For now, you should simply make a note that it occurs.

OTHER DIRECT VASODILATORS

There are several other agents that act directly on smooth muscle cells, resulting in vasodilation. For these other drugs, name recognition as vasodilators is the most important thing for you to focus on.

> Hydralazine and minoxidil directly relax arterioles.

The arteriole relaxation results in a decrease in blood pressure, but the exact mechanism of action of these drugs is not clear. The decrease in blood pressure leads to reflex tachycardia and increased cardiac output (not a desirable effect in a patient with limited cardiac reserve). These drugs will also increase plasma renin concentration. The reflex tachycardia can be blocked with β-blockers. Diuretics can be used to counter the sodium and water retention.

An aside: Minoxidil causes unwanted hair growth in patients receiving the drug for the treatment of hypertension. The drug is also marketed for topical treatment of baldness (under the trade name Rogaine).

> Fenoldopam is a dopamine agonist used for the acute treatment of severe hypertension.

Fenoldopam dilates renal and mesenteric vascular beds by acting as a selective DA_1 receptor agonist.

α- AND β-BLOCKERS

> The α_1 antagonists, such as PRAZOSIN, terazosin, and doxazosin, dilate arteries and veins.

Recall from the discussion of autonomic nervous system drugs that blood vessels are primarily under α receptor control. α Agonists cause vasoconstriction and α antagonists cause vasodilation. The α-blockers can be used to treat hypertension, but they are associated with postural hypotension, particularly after the first dose. Therefore, the use of α antagonists makes sense for the treatment of hypertension. The mixed α_1, β_1, and β_2 antagonist, labetalol, dilates blood vessels (α_1) without causing a reflex increase in heart rate (β_1).

> β-Blockers prevent sympathetic stimulation of the heart.

β-Blockers have some use in the treatment of hypertension. They decrease heart rate and cardiac output (β_1) and will decrease renin release (β_1). Similar to the ACE inhibitors, β-blockers may not be effective in lowering blood pressure in African American patients.

> β-Blockers may be particularly useful in patients with angina or those with migraines.

Some β-Blockers Used to Treat Hypertension

atenolol	β_1 antagonist
betaxolol	β_1 antagonist
bisoprolol	β_1 antagonist
metoprolol	β_1 antagonist
carvedilol	β_1 antagonist with α-blocking activity
labetalol	β_1 antagonist with α-blocking activity
nebivolol	β_1 antagonist plus nitric oxide–mediated activity
acebutolol	β_1 antagonist plus some sympathomimetic activity
esmolol	β_1 antagonist plus some sympathomimetic activity
penbutolol	β_1 antagonist plus some sympathomimetic activity
nadolol	β_1 and β_2 antagonist
PROPRANOLOL	β_1 and β_2 antagonist
timolol	β_1 and β_2 antagonist
pindolol	β_1 and β_2 antagonist plus some sympathomimetic activity

As you can see from the preceding box, both β_1 selective and nonselective blockers have been successfully used in hypertension.

CLONIDINE

Reduction of sympathetic outflow will result in a net decrease in blood pressure. Four drugs are active centrally: clonidine, methyldopa, (or α-methyldopa), guanabenz and guanfacine. Be sure you know their names and can identify these drugs as centrally active agents that reduce sympathetic outflow.

CLONIDINE is an α_2 agonist that reduces central sympathetic outflow.

These drugs decrease total peripheral resistance without changing cardiac output. As you might predict, these drugs have no direct effect on the kidney and can be used in patients with renal disease. The side effects of these drugs include drowsiness and dry mouth (sounds like anticholinergic actions to me). There are some differences in the mechanism of action of these compounds, but these differences are too far down on the trivia list to worry about now.

Drugs Used in Ischemic Heart Disease and Congestive Heart Failure

Ischemic Heart Disease
Congestive Heart Failure
Reduction of Cardiac Workload
Control of Excessive Fluid
Enhancement of Contractility
    Cardiac Glycosides
    Sympathomimetics
    Phosphodiesterase Inhibitors
    Ranolazine

ISCHEMIC HEART DISEASE

Ischemic heart disease is simply when the oxygen supply to the heart does not match the demand. Often this means that the coronary blood vessels have a reduced diameter limiting the blood flow to the heart.

> Pharmacologically, the treatment of coronary artery disease focuses on the reduction of myocardial oxygen demand.

To reduce myocardial oxygen demand β-blockers (Chapters 10 and 11) can be used to decrease heart rate and contractility. Calcium channel blockers (Chapter 11) reduce systemic vascular resistance and decrease myocardial contractility. Nitrates (Chapter 11) will produce venous dilation, which will decrease preload and decrease oxygen demand by the heart. Finally, antiplatelet drugs (Chapter 14), such as aspirin, will prevent thrombus formation in the coronary arteries. Lipid-lowering drugs (Chapter 15) have been shown to reduce the risk of heart attacks in patients with coronary artery disease.

Unstable angina is treated with nitroglycerin, antiplatelet, and anticoagulant drugs. Finally, acute myocardial infarction is treated with thrombolytic agents (Chapter 14).

CONGESTIVE HEART FAILURE

Heart failure occurs when the heart can no longer pump enough blood to meet the demands of the body. After removal or correction of the precipitating cause, further treatment of heart failure involves management of the symptoms. Standard treatment for hospitalized patients has been a loop diuretic (Chapter 11) with a vasodilator that is rapidly acting. Sometimes a drug that increases contractility is also added or used in place of the vasodilator.

> Treatment of heart failure is targeted toward decreasing cardiac workload, controlling excess fluid, and enhancing myocardial contractility.

REDUCTION OF CARDIAC WORKLOAD

> Angiotensin-converting enzyme (ACE) inhibitors lessen the symptoms of heart failure by reducing cardiac workload.

Achieving a reduction in cardiac workload can be as simple as reducing physical activity. Pharmacologically, vasodilator therapy can be used. ACE inhibitors (Chapter 11) are usually used in this instance. ACE inhibitors have been shown to improve symptoms, slow the progression of the heart failure, and prolong survival. The angiotensin II receptor antagonists are also used.

Other vasodilators also can be used to reduce the cardiac workload. Studies have shown that the combination of hydralazine and isosorbide dinitrate can produce improvement in patients with heart failure.

Nitroprusside is used in the treatment of acute heart failure because it reduces both preload and afterload without affecting contractility.

β-Blockers have also found a use in the treatment of heart failure. Although β-blockers can decrease contractility, the reduction in sympathetic stimulation can produce long-term benefits.

Nesiritide is a recombinant form of human B-type natriuretic peptide. B-type natriuretic peptide is a naturally occurring hormone produced by the ventricle. It produces natriuresis, diuresis and vasodilation by increasing intracellular cyclic guanosine monophosphate (cGMP) levels.

CONTROL OF EXCESSIVE FLUID

> Diuretics are almost always used to control excess fluid accumulation in heart failure.

Heart failure is associated with retention of sodium and water. Control of the excessive fluid accumulation can relieve symptoms. The first line of attack is to lower dietary intake of sodium. Diuretics are also used to relieve symptoms, but they do not stop the progression of the disease. All classes of diuretics are used; the choice depends on the clinical situation.

ENHANCEMENT OF CONTRACTILITY

CARDIAC GLYCOSIDES

The cardiac glycosides were originally isolated from the *Digitalis purpurea* plant; a fact that is reflected in their names—digitalis, digoxin, and digitoxin. The term *digitalis* is a general one that is usually used when referring to the drug digoxin.

> The cardiac glycosides (DIGOXIN and DIGITOXIN) improve myocardial contractility. They inhibit Na^+-K^+-ATPase.

These drugs inhibit sodium–potassium–ATPase and enhance release of intracellular calcium from the sarcoplasmic reticulum. This increase in intracellular calcium causes an increase in the force of contraction of the myocytes throughout the heart. In addition to their use in chronic heart failure, both digoxin and digitoxin will slow the ventricular rate in atrial flutter or fibrillation by increasing the sensitivity of the atrioventricular (AV) node to vagal stimulation. This makes them antiarrhythmic drugs as well (see Chapter 13).

> Digoxin has a *shorter* half-life, no (the ultimate *fewer*) metabolites, is *less* completely absorbed from the GI tract, and is *less* protein bound than digitoxin.

> The cardiac glycosides have a low therapeutic index.

As noted in Chapter 2, the therapeutic index is the LD_{50} divided by the ED_{50}. A low therapeutic index means that the plasma concentration that causes serious toxicity (that is, may be *fatal*) is only slightly higher than the therapeutic dose. The therapeutic index is between 1.6 and 2.5 for the cardiac glycosides. Toxicity of the cardiac glycosides is more common in patients with low serum potassium levels. This is quite important, because many patients with heart failure are taking "dig. and diuretics" (shorthand for digoxin and a diuretic).

Toxicity resulting from cardiac glycosides can be manifested by:

Arrhythmias

Anorexia, nausea, and diarrhea

Drowsiness and fatigue

Visual disturbances

Among these toxic effects, it is the arrhythmias that can be life-threatening.

SYMPATHOMIMETICS

These drugs were covered earlier in the autonomic nervous system section (see Chapter 9). Here is a quick review.

> DOBUTAMINE is a β_1 agonist. At moderate doses it increases contractility of the heart without changing blood pressure or heart rate.

Dobutamine is used to increase cardiac output in heart failure and can be used in the treatment of shock. Dobutamine has some α_1 and β_2 agonist effects that play a role in maintaining peripheral vascular resistance. It is only given intravenously, so its use is limited.

DOPAMINE has dopamine receptor agonist activity and, like dobutamine, is used in the treatment of acute heart failure.

In patients with impaired renal function, the use of dopamine (instead of dobutamine) may preserve renal blood flow and, as a result, renal function. Administration of dopamine is also limited to the IV route.

PHOSPHODIESTERASE INHIBITORS

Inamrinone (formerly amrinone) and milrinone inhibit the cyclic adenosine monophosphate (cAMP) phosphodiesterase in cardiac and vascular muscle. This results in a positive inotropic action as well as a vasodilatory effect. There is little increase in heart rate.

RANOLAZINE

Ranolazine is a relatively new drug (approved in 2006) for the treatment of chronic angina. Evidence suggests that ranolazine reduces calcium overload in the ischemic heart muscle cell through inhibition of the late sodium current (I_{Na}). Myocardial ischemia produces a cascade of complex ionic exchanges that can result in intracellular acidosis, excess cytosolic Ca^{2+}, myocardial cellular dysfunction, and, if sustained, cell injury and death. By inhibiting the excess calcium in the cells, cellular function would be maintained. This drug may not belong in this group of drugs that enhance contractility, but it's a good enough place for now.

Antiarrhythmic Drugs

Organization of Class
Class I Drugs (Sodium Channel Blockers)
Class II Drugs (β-Blockers)
Class III Drugs (Potassium Channel Blockers)
Class IV Drugs (Calcium Channel Blockers)
Other Antiarrhythmic Drugs
Drugs That Increase Heart Rate

ORGANIZATION OF CLASS

Arrhythmias, disturbances of the normal rhythm of the heart, occur when the electrical conduction systems malfunction. The malfunction could result in a change in heart rate, rhythm, impulse generation, or conduction of electrical signals through the heart muscle. Nonpharmacological approaches to arrhythmias include the use of pacemakers, implantable defibrillators, and ablation of an aberrant conduction pathway.

To understand the action and classification of the antiarrhythmic drugs, it is first necessary to understand the ionic movements that underlie the cardiac action potential (Figure 13–1). It is also good to remember the normal flow of electricity in the heart. What controls the rate? What controls the rhythm? What takes over in emergencies?

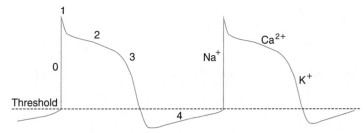

FIGURE 13–1 The cardiac action potential is shown. The action potential has been divided into phases (indicated on the left). The shape of the action potential is determined by the ions that are flowing during that phase (indicated on the right).

The antiarrhythmic agents are classified into four groups according to the part of the cardiac cycle they influence. This is a universal system, but it is not entirely accurate. Several drugs have more than one effect, and others do not fall into any of the four categories.

CLASS I DRUGS (SODIUM CHANNEL BLOCKERS)

> The class I drugs are essentially sodium channel blockers.

The class I drugs are characterized by their ability to block sodium entry into the cell during depolarization. This decreases the rate of rise of phase 0 of the action potential (Figure 13–2). These drugs also suppress automaticity of the Purkinje fibers and His bundle.

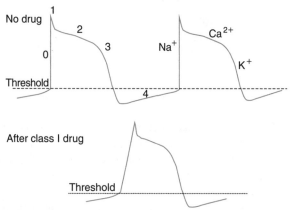

FIGURE 13–2 Class I antiarrhythmics block sodium entry into myocardial cells during depolarization. This decreases the rate of rise of phase 0.

The class I drugs have been further divided into three groups. The differences between classes A, B, and C are not of primary importance to beginning students of pharmacology; this information can be learned later. Class IA drugs slow the rate of rise of phase 0 and prolong the effective refractory period of the ventricle. Class IB drugs have less of an effect on phase 0, but shorten the action potential duration and refractory period of the Purkinje fibers. Class IC drugs have the greatest effect on the early depolarization and have less of an effect on the refractory period of the ventricle.

Class IA Drugs	Class IB Drugs	Class IC Drugs
PROCAINAMIDE	LIDOCAINE	flecainide
QUINIDINE	mexiletine	propafenone
disopyramide	phenytoin	
	tocainide	

Here we have a major stumbling block for pharmacology students. Notice that there appears to be little rhyme or reason in the names given to the class I drugs. If you have already covered these drugs in class, you may recognize some of the local anesthetics (procainamide and lidocaine). Many of these drug names do look a bit alike, because they end in "-cainide." Name recognition drilling will be most helpful with this group of drugs.

The names and overall mechanism of action are the most important points for you to know about the class I antiarrhythmics. Once you have mastered this information, you can add a few facts about some of the individual agents.

> The class IA drugs are useful in the treatment of atrial and ventricular arrhythmias.

These drugs—quinidine, procainamide, and disopyramide—are all-purpose antiarrhythmics. As you read through the uses and indications for these drugs, focus on the similarities. Later you can go back and consider the differences.

As you might guess from its name, quinidine is related to quinine. Both quinidine and quinine have antimalarial actions (see Chapter 34).

> The class IB drugs (LIDOCAINE is the *drug of choice*) are used for the treatment of ventricular arrhythmias (ventricular tachycardia, ventricular fibrillation, and ventricular ectopy).

The class IB drugs are much less effective in treating the atrial (supraventricular) arrhythmias than are the class IA drugs.

> The class IC agents are useful in suppressing ventricular arrhythmias.

Flecainide and propafenone are absorbed orally and are used for chronic suppression of ventricular arrhythmias (as opposed to acute treatment of patients with ventricular arrhythmias, which is the role of the class IB agents).

Moricizine is a class I antiarrhythmic agent with features of all three subclasses. It inhibits sodium influx through fast sodium channels in cardiac tissue in a use-dependent fashion. This means that the more the channel is used the more it is blocked.

CLASS II DRUGS (β-BLOCKERS)

> The class II antiarrhythmics are β-blockers.

The mechanism of action of these drugs, in terms of rhythm stabilization, is unknown. Use of the β-blockers results in cardiac membrane stabilization. Conduction through the sinoatrial (SA) and atrioventricular (AV) nodes is slowed and the refractory period is increased (Figure 13–3). A list of β-blockers is provided in Chapter 11.

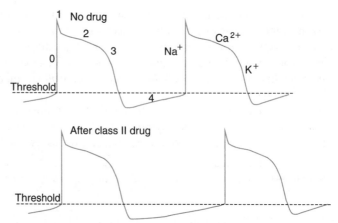

FIGURE 13–3 Class II antiarrhythmics increase the refractory period between action potentials.

> These drugs are particularly useful in suppressing the tachyarrhythmias that result from increased sympathetic activity.

> PROPRANOLOL is the β-blocker most commonly used to treat patients with arrhythmias.

CLASS III DRUGS (POTASSIUM CHANNEL BLOCKERS)

> The class III antiarrhythmics prolong repolarization. They are sometimes designated as potassium channel blockers.

These drugs show complex pharmacological properties. They are classified together because they all prolong the duration of the action potential without altering phase 0 depolarization or the resting membrane potential (Figure 13–4).

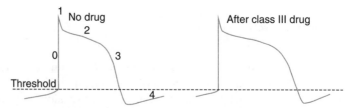

FIGURE 13–4 Class III antiarrhythmics prolong the duration of the action potential without altering phase 0 depolarization or the resting membrane potential.

Class III Drugs

BRETYLIUM
AMIODARONE
dronedarone
dofetilide
ibutilide
sotalol

It is probably wise to include these drug names in your name recognition list. Note, however, that many books do not include sotalol here. You should check your textbook or lecture notes.

> The class III agents are useful in treating intractable ventricular arrhythmias.

Amiodarone has largely replaced lidocaine in situations of cardiac arrest and is effective in the treatment and prevention of ventricular fibrillation and ventricular tachycardia. However, dofetilide is used to convert atrial fibrillation and maintain sinus rhythm after cardioversion. So you can see, the general rules don't always apply. Dronedarone is an analogue of amiodarone without the iodine. It appears to be less toxic than amiodarone.

Not all class III drugs block potassium currents. Ibutilide promotes the influx of sodium through slow inward sodium channels, resulting in a prolongation of the action potential. This results in slowing of the heart rate and conduction through the AV node. Ibutilide is indicated for the conversion of atrial fibrillation or flutter to normal sinus rhythm.

CLASS IV DRUGS (CALCIUM CHANNEL BLOCKERS)

> The class IV antiarrhythmics are the calcium channel blockers. These drugs slow conduction through the AV node and increase the effective refractory period in the AV node.

These actions may terminate reentrant arrhythmias that require the AV node for conduction. A list of calcium channel blockers is provided in Chapter 12. Some calcium channel blockers have a greater effect on the heart than on the vascular smooth muscle; the effects of others are just the opposite.

These drugs block the slow inward calcium current during phases 0 and 2 of the cardiac cycle. By slowing the inward calcium current, these drugs slow conduction and prolong the effective refractory period, especially in the AV node.

> The calcium channel blockers are more effective against atrial than ventricular arrhythmias.

The side effects of these drugs are the result of their other actions, such as vasodilation. This should come as no surprise.

OTHER ANTIARRHYTHMIC DRUGS

As previously noted, there are a number of drugs that do not neatly fall into the four classes of antiarrhythmics. Among these other antiarrhythmic drugs are adenosine and the cardiac glycosides (digoxin).

> ADENOSINE is highly effective in terminating paroxysmal supraventricular tachycardia.

Adenosine is given intravenously and has an exceedingly short half-life (in seconds). It depresses AV and sinus node activity. Because the most common form of paroxysmal supraventricular tachycardia involves a reentrant pathway, adenosine is effective in terminating the arrhythmia.

> DIGOXIN is used to control the ventricular rate in atrial fibrillation or flutter.

Digoxin slows conduction through the AV node and increases the refractory period of the AV node. This decreases the number and frequency of impulses that pass from the atria into the ventricles. That's important when the atria are out of control, as in flutter or fibrillation.

DRUGS THAT INCREASE HEART RATE

> Drugs that can be used to increase heart rate include ATROPINE, ISOPROTERENOL, and EPINEPHRINE.

These drugs are used to treat bradycardia. Blocking the parasympathetic system (which tries to slow the heart) with atropine (a muscarinic antagonist) will increase the heart rate. For you trivia buffs, a total dose of 3 mg of atropine will produce complete blockade of vagal activity. Sympathetic agonists will also increase heart rate by directly stimulating the β receptors in the heart. The increase in heart rate and contractility can worsen ischemia in a patient whose heart is at risk.

Drugs That Affect Blood

- Organization of Class
- Antiplatelet Agents
- Anticoagulants
- Thrombolytic Drugs
- Phosphodiesterase Inhibitors
- Drugs Used in the Treatment of Anemia

ORGANIZATION OF CLASS

The process of hemostasis consists of three phases: vascular, platelet, and coagulation (Figure 14–1). The fibrinolytic phase that follows prevents the clotting process from spreading out of control beyond the site of injury. It may be helpful at this point to review the hemostatic mechanisms in your physiology textbook.

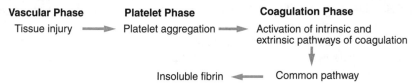

FIGURE 14–1 Hemostasis consists of three phases: vascular, platelet, and coagulation. The end result of these phases is the formation of fibrin.

Platelets respond to tissue injury by adhering to the site of injury; they then release granules containing chemical mediators that promote aggregation. Factors released by platelets and the injured tissue cause activation of the coagulation cascade. This results in the formation of thrombin, which in turn converts fibrinogen to fibrin. The subsequent cross-linking of the fibrin strands stabilizes the clot.

Drugs are available that interfere with the platelet and coagulation phases of the initial response to tissue injury. As we review the drugs that prevent clots and those that lyse clots, the drugs that can function as antidotes will be mentioned. Finally, we'll consider drugs used to treat anemia.

ANTIPLATELET AGENTS

Platelet aggregation inhibitors decrease the formation of chemical signals that promote platelet aggregation. Drugs that inhibit platelet function are administered for the relatively specific *prophylaxis* of arterial thrombosis and during management of heart attacks (myocardial infarction). Upon stimulation, platelets synthesize thromboxane A$_2$ (TXA$_2$). TXA$_2$ is considered to be a specific stimulus for aggregation.

> Nonsteroidal anti-inflammatory drugs (NSAIDs), including aspirin, inhibit platelet aggregation and prolong bleeding time.

Antiplatelet Drugs

NSAIDs, including aspirin	**IIB/IIIA receptor antagonists**
anagrelide	abciximab
clopidogrel	eptifibatide
dipyridamole	tirofiban
prasugrel	
ridogrel	
ticlopidine	

NSAIDs will be considered in more detail in Chapter 43. These agents inhibit cyclooxygenase. In platelets, this inhibits the formation of TXA$_2$ (a thromboxane). TXA$_2$ is a potent inducer of platelet aggregation. Aspirin acetylates cyclooxygenase-1 (COX-1) effectively inhibiting platelet aggregation for 5-7 days.

Dipyridamole decreases platelet adhesion to damaged endothelium, but does not alter bleeding time. Dipyridamole inhibits platelet uptake of adenosine. It is usually used in combination with aspirin or warfarin.

Ticlopidine and clopidogrel inhibit platelet aggregation and prolong bleeding time. They work by inactivating the platelet P2Y12 (ADP) receptor, thus having a prolonged action.

> Platelet glycoprotein IIb/IIIa receptor antagonists prevent platelet aggregation by blocking the binding of fibrinogen and von Willebrand factor to the glycoprotein IIb/IIIa receptor on the surface of the platelet.

The glycoprotein receptor, known as the IIb/IIIa receptor, is critical for platelet aggregation. Fibrinogen molecules bind to these receptors and form bridges between adjacent platelets, allowing them to aggregate. Abciximab is a monoclonal antibody to the receptor, eptifibatide and tirofiban are platelet IIb/IIIa receptor antagonists. All of these drugs increase the risk of bleeding, particularly at the site of arterial access.

Ridogrel inhibits the arachidonic acid pathway at two sites. It is an inhibitor of TXA$_2$ synthase, blocking TXA$_2$ formation, and is also a prostaglandin endoperoxide receptor antagonist.

A slightly different anti-platelet drug is anagrelide. Anagrelide will inhibit platelet aggregation, but also reduces platelet count, most likely by inhibiting megakaryocyte development in the late, postmitotic stage. It can be used in the treatment of essential thrombocythemia.

ANTICOAGULANTS

Anticoagulant drugs inhibit the development and enlargement of clots. It should be obvious from the name of the group that the drugs act by interfering with the coagulation phase of hemostasis. These drugs are divided into two to four groups in various books. The simplest organization is "heparin and the others". The others are orally active and include warfarin and dicumarol. A more complete organization is (1) the heparin class, including the parenteral (heparin and low-molecular-weight heparins) and orally administered agents (warfarin and dicumarol), (2) direct thrombin inhibitors, and (3) others.

Anticoagulant Drugs

Heparin and LMWH	Thrombin inhibitors
HEPARIN	hirudin
ardeparin	argatroban
dalteparin	bivalirudin
danaparoid	dabigatran
enoxaparin	desirudin
tinzaparin	lepirudin
Oral anticoagulants	Others
warfarin	fondaparinux
dicumarol	drotrecogin alfa

> The major side effect of all of the anticoagulants is hemorrhage.

The preceding statement should be intuitive, but it warrants a mention. Anticoagulant therapy provides prophylaxis against venous and arterial thrombosis. These drugs cannot dissolve clots that have already formed, but they may prevent or slow extension of an existing clot. They are useful in preventing deep vein thrombosis and pulmonary embolism. Anticoagulation therapy in patients with atrial fibrillation has reduced the risk of systemic embolism and stroke.

> HEPARIN interferes with clotting factor activation in both the intrinsic and extrinsic pathway.

The principal anticoagulant actions of heparin are a result of its binding to antithrombin III. Heparin also inactivates factors IIa, IXa, Xa, XIa, XIIa, and XIIIa and neutralizes tissue thromboplastin (factor III). The low-molecular-weight heparins are oligosaccharides extracted from heparin. These agents have larger anti-Xa to anti-IIa activity ratios than heparin, which permits them to be used at lower doses. In addition, the low-molecular-weight heparins have greater bioavailability after subcutaneous injection and have a longer half-life than heparin.

> PROTAMINE is a specific heparin antagonist that can be used to treat heparin-induced hemorrhage.

Protamines are basic proteins that have a high affinity for the negatively charged heparin. The binding of protamine and heparin is immediate and results in an inert complex.

> Warfarin, a vitamin K antagonist, is the oral anticoagulant of choice.

Before they can participate in the clotting process, several of the protein coagulation factors require vitamin K for their activation. The oral anticoagulants interfere with this action of vitamin K. Therefore, the oral anticoagulants delay activation of new coagulation factors (Figure 14–2). They do not affect the factors that have already been activated. This means there is a delay in the onset of action of the oral anticoagulants. The oral anticoagulants are used when long-term therapy is indicated.

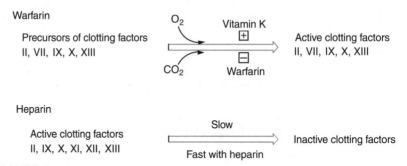

FIGURE 14–2 As a visual reminder, this figure diagrams the processes by which warfarin blocks activation of clotting factors and heparin speeds the inactivation of clotting factors.

> Administration of vitamin K can overcome the anticoagulant effects of the oral agents, but the effect takes about 24 hours.

The time it takes for vitamin K to overcome the anticoagulant effects of the oral agents is also directly related to the mechanism of action. It takes time to make new coagulation factors.

> There are a large number of drug interactions with the oral anticoagulants.

There are many drugs that both increase and decrease the effect of the oral anticoagulants. It is not possible to memorize them all. The important thing for now is to remember that there are many drug interactions.

There are some newer anticoagulant drugs that act on specific coagulation factors. Fondaparinux is a synthetic compound that binds to antithrombin causing it to inhibit factor Xa. Drotrecogin alfa is a recombinant form of human activated protein C and inhibits factors Va and VIIIa. Drotrecogin alfa may also have anti-inflammatory effects and has been shown to increase survival in patients with sepsis.

> Direct thrombin inhibitors are also effective anticoagulants.

Thrombin plays a number of critical roles in coagulation. The first direct thrombin inhibitor, hirudin, was derived from the medicinal leech. Others, including bivalirudin, desirudin, lepirudin, are recombinant forms of the natural hirudin.

THROMBOLYTIC DRUGS

Thrombolytic Drugs

STREPTOKINASE	reteplase
alteplase	t-PA
anistreplase	tenecteplase
lanoteplase	urokinase

> Anticoagulant and antiplatelet drugs are administered to prevent the formation or extension of clots. Thrombolytic drugs are used to lyse already formed clots.

This is an important distinction for the clinical use of these drugs. Fibrinolysis is the process of breaking down the fibrin that holds the clot together. Fibrinolysis is initiated by the activation of plasminogen to plasmin. The plasmin then catalyzes the degradation of fibrin. The activation of plasminogen is normally initiated by plasminogen activators (straightforward so far?).

> The thrombolytic drugs are plasminogen activators.

There are currently two generations of plasminogen activators, first and second. The first-generation drugs (including streptokinase and urokinase) convert all plasminogen to plasmin throughout the plasma. The second-generation drugs (including tissue plasminogen activator, or t-PA) selectively activate plasminogen that is bound to fibrin. This is supposed to reduce the side effects of the drug by targeting the site of action.

> Clot dissolution and reperfusion are more likely if therapy is initiated early after clot formation. Clots become more difficult to lyse as they age.

Thrombolytic drugs have been shown to lyse clots in arteries and veins and to reestablish tissue perfusion. They are used in the management of pulmonary embolism, deep vein thrombosis, and arterial thromboembolism. They have proven to be particularly useful in acute heart attacks caused by a clot in a coronary artery.

> The main side effect of the thrombolytic drugs is bleeding.

This statement should not come as a surprise to you.

> STREPTOKINASE is a foreign protein and is antigenic. t-PA is not antigenic.

The antigenicity of streptokinase (a result of its bacterial origin), produces one of the side effects of this drug: an allergic–anaphylactic reaction. Patients may also develop antibodies to streptokinase and inactivate it. These reactions are less likely to occur after t-PA administration, because t-PA is of human origin (produced through recombinant DNA technology).

Recombinant forms of t-PA, including reteplase, alteplase, and lanoteplase, are now available. They differ from t-PA in time for onset of action and duration of action.

Direct thrombin inhibitors have been studied for prophylaxis against, and treatment of, thromboembolism. One such drug is ximelagatran, which is a prodrug for melagatran, which is a reversible inhibitor of both free and clot-bound thrombin. It is not available in the United States.

PHOSPHODIESTERASE INHIBITORS

> Phosphodiesterase III inhibitors (pentoxifylline and cilostazol) are used to treat intermittent claudication.

Intermittent claudication is a symptom of peripheral arterial disease and often causes debilitating pain, aches, and cramps in the legs that reduce a person's ability to walk. These agents target multiple processes related to peripheral circulation, including inhibition of platelet aggregation, and cause vasodilation.

DRUGS USED IN THE TREATMENT OF ANEMIA

Anemia is defined as a plasma hemoglobin level that is below normal. It can reflect decreased numbers of circulating red blood cells or an abnormally low total hemoglobin content. There are many causes of anemia. Before treatment, the cause needs to be determined.

Drugs Used to Treat Anemia

ERYTHROPOIETIN

IRON

cyanocobalamin (vitamin B_{12})

epoetin alfa, darbepoetin alfa

folic acid

Iron salts, such as ferrous sulfate, are used as iron supplements to treat iron deficiency anemia.

Folic acid and vitamin B_{12} are used to treat anemias caused by deficiencies of these vitamins.

Erythropoietin is synthesized in the kidney in response to hypoxia or anemia. It then stimulates erythropoiesis (red cell proliferation).

Epoetin alfa and darbepoetin alfa are human recombinant erythropoietins.

Human erythropoietin is used in the treatment of anemia associated with end-stage renal failure.

15 Lipid-Lowering Drugs

Organization of Class
Additional Explanation of Mechanisms

ORGANIZATION OF CLASS

Coronary artery disease, heart attacks, and strokes have been shown to be correlated with plasma levels of serum cholesterol and lipoprotein particles. Therefore, there has been increased interest in lowering the cholesterol and lipoprotein levels in at-risk patients by diet or by pharmacological intervention.

Drugs used in the treatment of elevated serum lipids (hyperlipidemias) are targeted to decrease production of lipoprotein or cholesterol, increase degradation of a lipoprotein, or increase removal of cholesterol from the body.

The lipoproteins are proteins that bind and transport fats, such as lipids and triglycerides, in the blood. They are classified according to lipid and protein content, transport function, and mechanism of lipid delivery. The high-density lipoproteins (HDL) are often referred to as the "good cholesterol" in contrast to the low- and very-low-density lipoproteins (LDL and VLDL), the "bad cholesterol."

The most important facts about the relatively few drugs in this class are the mechanisms of action. Practically speaking, taste, dose, and cost are also important considerations.

Drugs	Mechanism
LOVASTATIN	Inhibit HMG-CoA reductase
atorvastatin	
cerivastatin	
fluvastatin	
pitavastatin	
pravastatin	
rosuvastatin	
simvastatin	

(Continued)

Drugs	Mechanism
CHOLESTYRAMINE	Bile acid–binding resins
colesevelam	
colestipol	
EZETIMIBE	Inhibits absorption of cholesterol
niacin	?
bezafibrate	Increase lipoprotein lipase activity
clofibrate	
fenofibrate	
gemfibrozil	

First, compare the list of drugs in the preceding box with that in your text-book or class handouts and add or delete drugs as needed. Next, compare the mechanisms of action noted here to those in your textbook or handouts. Some of these mechanisms are not entirely worked out so there may be discrepancies. Don't let that throw you off.

Basically, this box summarizes the most important things to know. If there is too much information here for you to absorb at one sitting, start by learning the two bile-binding resins and the drugs that inhibit HMG-CoA reductase (identified by their common ending of "-statin"). The rest of the drugs alter metabolism of lipoproteins. If you already have a good grasp of this content, you can skip the rest of this chapter.

ADDITIONAL EXPLANATION OF MECHANISMS

HMG-CoA reductase inhibitors are the first-choice drugs for treatment of most patients with hypercholesterolemia. These drugs, referred to generally as "-statins," contain structural analogues of 3-hydroxy-3-methylglutarate (HMG), which is a precursor of cholesterol. They inhibit HMG-CoA reductase, the enzyme that controls the rate-limiting step in cholesterol synthesis. This depletes intracellular cholesterol. The cell then looks to the extracellular space for the cholesterol it needs. The result is a lowering of the plasma cholesterol and LDL levels. Statins also improve endothelial function, decrease platelet aggregation and reduce inflammation. These drugs must be taken indefinitely as cholesterol levels will return to predrug levels within weeks of stopping the statin. The first side effect to know is myalgia, which is fairly common.

The bile-binding resins (cholestyramine, colestipol, and colesevelam) are anion exchange resins that bind negatively charged bile acids in the small intestine. The resins are not absorbed and are not metabolized. The resin–bile acid complex is excreted in the feces (Figure 15–1). The body compensates for the reduction in bile acids by converting cholesterol to bile acids, thus effectively lowering the cholesterol levels. Because of the mechanism of action, it should seem reasonable to you that these resins may also affect the absorption of other drugs and the fat-soluble vitamins. A new drug, ezetimibe, inhibits the absorption of dietary and biliary cholesterol from the small intestine without working through the bile acids. It does not affect triglyceride absorption.

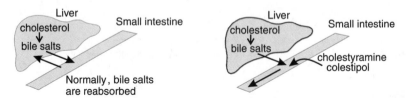

FIGURE 15-1 Normally, bile acids are secreted into the small intestine and then reabsorbed almost completely. Cholestyramine and colestipol bind to the bile acids in the small intestine and prevent their reabsorption. This causes the liver to use cholesterol to make more bile acids.

Niacin lowers both plasma cholesterol and triglyceride levels. The lipid-lowering effects are the result of decreased hepatic secretion of VLDL. This appears to be due to decreased triglyceride synthesis.

Gemfibrozil, fenofibrate, and clofibrate—the "-fibrates"—are used mainly to lower triglycerides and increase HDL cholesterol.

Another strategy actively being explored to reduce the risk of coronary artery disease is inhibition of the cholesteryl ester transfer protein (CETP). This protein is a plasma glycoprotein that facilitates the transfer of cholesteryl esters from HDL cholesterol to apolipoprotein B–containing lipoproteins. Although that torcetrapib (a CETP inhibitor) will increase HDL levels, while decreasing LDL levels, it failed to reduce atheroselerotic plaque burden in a large clinical trial.

PART IV Drugs That Act on the Central Nervous System

CHAPTER 16:   Drugs Used in Dementia   91

CHAPTER 17:   Anxiolytic and Hypnotic Drugs   93

CHAPTER 18:   Drugs Used in Mood Disorders   100

CHAPTER 19:   Antipsychotics or Neuroleptics   106

CHAPTER 20:   Drugs Used in Parkinson Disease   110

CHAPTER 21:   Antiepileptic Drugs   113

CHAPTER 22:   Narcotics (Opiates)   117

CHAPTER 23:   General Anesthetics   122

CHAPTER 24:   Local Anesthetics   126

Drugs Used in Dementia

Organization of Class
Cholinesterase Inhibitors
NMDA Blocker

ORGANIZATION OF CLASS

Dementia, including Alzheimer disease, has been found to involve a number of systems in the brain. There is evidence for a decrease in markers of cholinergic neuron activity *and* for changes in brain glutamate, dopamine, norepinephrine, serotonin, and somatostatin. Eventually, cholinergic neurons die or are destroyed. Treatment has focused on increasing the amount of acetylcholine in the synapse by inhibiting the breakdown of acetylcholine.

> None of the drugs available for dementia alter the underlying pathology. They produce only a marginal improvement in symptoms.

Cholinesterase inhibitors	NMDA antagonist
DONEPEZIL	MEMANTINE
galantamine	
rivastigmine	
tacrine	

CHOLINESTERASE INHIBITORS

Acetylcholinesterase is the enzyme the breaks down synaptically released acetylcholine (Chapter 7). Other cholinesterase inhibitors have been used as nerve gases or in the treatment of myasthenia gravis. The group of cholinesterases used in dementia appears to have a selectivity for the brain enzyme and, therefore, have fewer systemic side effects than you would predict. The cholinesterase inhibitors are used in mild to moderate disease.

Of the drugs currently available, tacrine is the oldest, but has limited use. Galantamine has some additional agonist activity at nicotinic receptors to enhance release of acetylcholine.

NMDA BLOCKER

> Memantine is a noncompetitive antagonist at the NMDA subtype of glutamate receptor.

The mechanism of action of memantine in dementia is not well understood. NMDA receptors are involved in learning and memory and blocking these receptors should block memory formation. NMDA receptors also allow calcium influx into neurons and have been implicated in excitotoxicity in the presence of excess glutamate. Memantine is a low-affinity blocker of the channel, so it is thought that memantine can block excess calcium influx, but can't block the physiological actions of glutamate involved in learning.

Memantine appears to be effective in patients on cholinesterase inhibitors.

Anxiolytic and Hypnotic Drugs

Tolerance and Dependence
Organization of Class
Barbiturates
Benzodiazepines
Buspirone
Benzodiazepine Receptor Agonists
Melatonin Receptor Agonist

TOLERANCE AND DEPENDENCE

Before we move on to the central nervous system (CNS) sedatives and narcotics, we need to clarify a few terms and definitions.

> Tolerance is a physiological state characterized by a reduced drug effect with repeated use of the drug. Higher doses are needed to produce the same effect.

Essentially, tolerance is a state of reduced effectiveness. The term does not give any indication of the mechanism involved. Tolerance could be the result of increased elimination of a drug or of reduced effectiveness of drug–receptor interaction. For some drugs, tolerance develops to one effect of the drug and not to other effects. For example, with the narcotics, tolerance is seen to the analgesic effect, but less tolerance develops to the respiratory depression.

> Cross-tolerance means that individuals tolerant to one drug will be tolerant to other drugs in the same class, but not to drugs in other classes.

A person who is tolerant to the sedative effects of one barbiturate will be tolerant to the effect of all the barbiturates (a situation termed cross-tolerance). However, that person will not be tolerant to the sedative effects of opiates.

> Dependence is characterized by signs and symptoms of withdrawal when drug levels fall.

Dependence can be physical, in which case the person has physical signs of withdrawal, or it can be psychological, in which case the person has psychological signs of withdrawal. There is something called cross-dependence, which is similar to cross-tolerance.

ORGANIZATION OF CLASS

Drugs that are classified as anxiolytics and hypnotics are used for a variety of purposes, including treatment of anxiety and epilepsy, sleep induction, and anesthesia. They are often called sedative-hypnotics or just anxiolytics.

> Cross-tolerance and cross-dependence occur between all of the CNS sedatives, including the barbiturates, benzodiazepines, and ethanol.

This is an important feature of all the drugs in this class.

These drugs are generally classified by chemical structure. The two largest groups of drugs are the barbiturates and benzodiazepines. There are a relatively large number of drugs in both of these groups, but (thankfully) their names are generally recognizable. The barbiturates are no longer used to treat anxiety, but it is easier to learn them in this context.

Barbiturates	Benzodiazepines	Others	NBBRAs
PHENOBARBITAL	ALPRAZOLAM	BUSPIRONE	zaleplon
THIOPENTAL	DIAZEPAM	chloral hydrate	zolpidem
amobarbital	LORAZEPAM	ramelteon	eszopiclone
methohexital	clonazepam		
pentobarbital	clorazepate		
secobarbital	flurazepam		
	oxazepam		
	quazepam		
	temazepam		
	triazolam		

Notice that the barbiturates all end in "-tal" and all *except* thiopental and methohexital end in "-barbital." The benzodiazepines, for the most part, end in "-pam" or "-lam." The notable exception here is chlordiazepoxide. This nomenclature makes it easy to succeed at name recognition.

All of these drugs reduce anxiety at low doses and produce sedation at slightly higher doses (Figure 17–1). Most induce sleep (hypnosis); thus, the name sedative-hypnotics. At higher doses the barbiturates produce some degree of anesthesia, and at even higher doses, produce medullary depression and death.

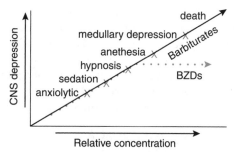

FIGURE 17–1 This graph schematizes the effects of the benzodiazepines (BZDs) and barbiturates. Notice that the effects of the barbiturates continue up the line of CNS depression to death, whereas the benzodiazepines veer off after hypnosis.

BARBITURATES

> Barbiturates enhance the function of γ-aminobutyric acid (GABA) in the CNS.

Barbiturates both enhance GABA responses and mimic GABA by opening the chloride channel in the absence of GABA. The net result of both actions is an increase in inhibition in the CNS.

> Barbiturates will
> 1. Produce sedation, hypnosis, coma, and *death*
> 2. Suppress respiration (overdose can lead to *death*)
> 3. Induce the liver P-450 system

All the barbiturates suppress respiration by inhibiting the hypoxic and CO_2 response of the chemoreceptors. This means that a slight increase in the CO_2 content of the blood does not result in an increase in respirations when the patient has taken barbiturates.

> Any other drug that is metabolized by the P-450 system will be altered by the presence of barbiturates.

All the barbiturates are metabolized by the liver and *all* induce the cytochrome P-450 microsomal enzymes. Thus, there is a long list of drug interactions for the barbiturates.

> The selection of a particular barbiturate depends on the duration of action of the agent, which in turn depends on its lipid solubility.

The barbiturates are classified according to their duration of action. Thiopental is an ultra-short-acting agent (minutes); pentobarbital, secobarbital, and amobarbital are short-acting agents (hours); and phenobarbital is a long-acting agent (days). Thiopental (ultra-short-acting) is highly lipid soluble. After administration, it rapidly enters the brain and then is redistributed into other body tissues and eventually into fat. As it is redistributed the concentration in the brain drops below effective levels. Therefore, the duration of action of thiopental is very short.

Do not try to memorize the duration of action of the barbiturates. Learn the few that are clinically useful today. Thiopental and methohexital, the ultra-short-acting barbiturates, are used in anesthesia (see Chapter 23). The long-duration barbiturate phenobarbital is used to treat epilepsy (see Chapter 21).

> Symptoms of withdrawal in a person dependent on barbiturates include anxiety, nausea and vomiting, hypotension, seizures, and psychosis. Cardiovascular collapse may develop, leading to *death*.

Physical dependence on barbiturates develops with chronic use. The symptoms of barbiturate withdrawal can be quite serious and even *fatal*.

BENZODIAZEPINES

> Benzodiazepines bind to a specific site associated with the GABA$_A$ receptor, which results in increased inhibition.

Binding of benzodiazepines to this specific site enhances the affinity of GABA receptors for GABA, resulting in more frequent opening of the chloride channels. The increased influx of chloride causes hyperpolarization and increased inhibition.

All benzodiazepines reduce anxiety and produce sedation. In contrast to the barbiturates, the benzodiazepines reduce anxiety at doses that do not produce sedation. Some agents are used as antiepileptic agents and some are used in the induction of anesthesia. Duration of action and pharmacokinetic properties are important considerations in selecting the drug to be used.

> Most benzodiazepines are metabolized in the liver to active metabolites. In general the metabolites have slower elimination rates than the parent compound.

It is not necessary to memorize a metabolism scheme for the benzodiazepines. However, as a glance at Figure 17–2 will show, many of the agents in this class appear to be interrelated.

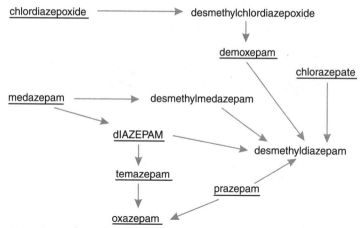

FIGURE 17–2 The metabolism and interrelationship of many of the benzodiazepines are shown in this figure. The compounds that are available pharmacological preparations are underlined.

A few benzodiazepines are *not* extensively metabolized. They tend to have shorter half-lives.

This issue of elimination half-life for the benzodiazepines can be confusing. It may not always be clear whether a textbook is referring to the half-life of the parent compound only or the total half-life of the parent plus the active metabolites.

> Elimination half-life is not the same as duration of action for the benzodiazepines.

The elimination half-life is determined by the rate of liver metabolism or renal excretion, or both. In other words, the half-life measures the time that the drug is present in the body. It gives no indication about the time the drug is present at the GABA receptors in the brain, which represents the duration of action. A drug that is hidden in a fat pad may not be metabolized by the liver microsomal enzymes for several days. This drug would have a very long elimination half-live and a short duration of action, because it has no action on the brain while hidden in fat.

> Physical and psychological dependence to benzodiazepines can occur.

Withdrawal from benzodiazepines can appear as confusion, anxiety, agitation, and restlessness. Benzodiazepines with short half-lives induce more abrupt and severe withdrawal reactions than do drugs with longer half-lives.

> FLUMAZENIL is a benzodiazepine antagonist.

Flumazenil can be used to reverse the sedative effects of benzodiazepines after anesthesia or after overdose with benzodiazepines.

It may be helpful to add some specific facts about the use of individual agents to the general knowledge we have reviewed so far.

> Some specific benzodiazepines have special uses. DIAZEPAM and LORAZEPAM are used in the treatment of status epilepticus. CHLORDIAZEPOXIDE is used in cases of alcohol withdrawal.

Over the years different benzodiazepines have been preferred for the treatment of anxiety. The recent favorite has been alprazolam. You can use the "a" at the beginning of its name to help you remember its use in *a*nxiety.

BUSPIRONE

> BUSPIRONE is a non-benzodiazepine that is used to treat generalized anxiety disorder.

Buspirone is relatively nonsedating and has few CNS side effects. It is an agonist at 5-HT_{1A} receptors and also has activity at 5-HT_{2A} and dopamine (D_2) receptors. Buspirone does not produce dependence. Because it does not act at the GABA receptor–chloride channel, buspirone is not recommended for the treatment of withdrawal from benzodiazepines.

It is interesting to compare the benzodiazepines with buspirone. Benzodiazepines have an effect after a single dose and need days to achieve a full therapeutic effect, whereas buspirone does not have an effect with a single dose and needs weeks to achieve a full therapeutic effect.

BENZODIAZEPINE RECEPTOR AGONISTS

Normally it's great when a class of drugs is named according to the mechanism of action, but in this case it's a mouthful. Zaleplon, zolpidem, and eszopiclone are known as non-benzodiazepine benzodiazepine receptor agonists (NBBRAs). In other words, they are not structurally related to benzodiazepines (Fig. 17-3), but they are agonists at the benzodiazepine receptor. All three drugs will shorten the time it takes to fall asleep. These drugs are used for short-term treatment of insomnia.

MELATONIN RECEPTOR AGONIST

Ramelteon is a melatonin receptor agonist that will help one fall asleep 7-16 minutes faster.

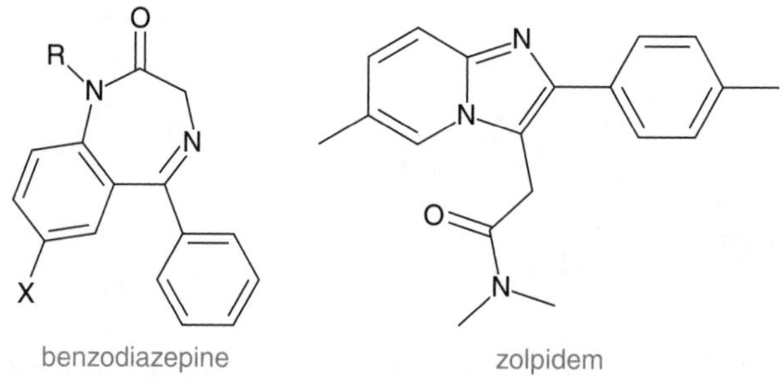

benzodiazepine   zolpidem

FIGURE 17-3 On the left is the general structure of a benzodiazepine. On the right is a non-benzodiazepine benzodiazepine agonist—zolpidem. As you can see the structures are quite different.

18 Drugs Used in Mood Disorders

Organization of Antidepressants

Serotonin-Specific Reuptake Inhibitors (SSRIs)

Serotonin/Norepinephrine Reuptake Inhibitors (SNRIs)

Heterocyclics/TCAs

Monoamine Oxidase (MAO) Inhibitors

Other Antidepressants

Drugs Used in Bipolar Disorder

ORGANIZATION OF CLASS

All of the antidepressant drugs increase the concentration of norepinephrine or serotonin in the synaptic cleft. In most cases, they do this by inhibiting the reuptake of the neurotransmitters. Remember that reuptake is the major route for termination of action of these neurotransmitters. Other drugs block their metabolic degradation or increase their release.

It is most logical to divide the antidepressants into five groups. Three groups are named according to their mechanism of action. Therefore, if you can remember the name of the group, you have already learned an important fact about each drug in the group. One group, the heterocyclics, consists mostly of tricyclic compounds (tricyclic antidepressants—TCA). They are grouped together mainly on the basis of structure, but they also have similar actions and side effects.

The trouble most students seem to have with these drugs is with their names. As you can see from the following table, the names of these drugs give no clues to their class. This is one instance where name recognition becomes very important for examination preparation. You may know everything about the monoamine oxidase (MAO) inhibitors, but if you do not recognize that tranylcypromine belongs in that group you may not be able to answer a question about this drug.

SSRIs	SNRIs	Heterocyclics	MAO Inhibitors	Others
FLUOEXTINE	desvenlafaxine	DESIPRAMINE	isocarboxazid	BUPROPION
citalopram	duloxetine	IMIPRAMINE	phenelzine	mirtazapine
escitalopram	milnacipran	amitriptyline	tranylcypromine	nefazodone
fluvoxamine	venlafaxine	doxepin		trazodone
paroxetine		maprotiline		
reboxetine		nortriptyline		
sertraline				

Learn what you can about each class of antidepressant and then be sure that you know the names of the drugs in each class.

SEROTONIN-SPECIFIC REUPTAKE INHIBITORS (SSRIs)

> SSRIs are antidepressants that block the reuptake of serotonin.

These drugs block the reuptake of serotonin, without affecting reuptake of norepinephrine or dopamine. Therefore, they are referred to as serotonin-specific reuptake inhibitors or selective serotonin reuptake inhibitors. Either name gives you the abbreviation SSRI. It is currently believed that the mechanism by which these drugs alleviate depression is by their blockade of the reuptake of serotonin. This may seem self-evident. If so, then it should be easy for you to remember. It takes several weeks of treatment with SSRIs to achieve a full therapeutic effect and there is no evidence that one SSRI is more effective than any other.

The initial treatment of choice for most patients is an SSRI. Drugs in this class are effective in a wide range of disorders in addition to depression. SSRIs have efficacy in eating disorders, panic disorder, obsessive compulsive disorder, and borderline personality disorder.

> SSRIs are not cholinergic antagonists or α-blockers.

SSRIs are essentially devoid of agonist or antagonist activity at any neurotransmitter receptor. Sexual dysfunction is a side effect of the drugs in this class. Severe withdrawal symptoms can occur if the SSRI is stopped abruptly.

SEROTONIN/NOREPINEPHRINE REUPTAKE INHIBITORS (SNRIs)

> Venlafaxine is an effective antidepressant that blocks reuptake of both serotonin and norepinephrine.

The SNRIs block reuptake of both serotonin and norepinephrine, hence the name of the class. Desvenlafaxine is an active metabolite of venlafaxine, but with no clinical advantage over the parent compound. Duloxetine is also approved for the treatment of diabetic neuropathy and fibromyalgia. Some clinicians feel that the SNRIs have fewer side effects than the SSRIs. However, the side effects with SNRIs are reported to be similar to that with SSRIs. SNRIs can cause a dose-dependent increase in blood pressure, presumably due to blocking reuptake of norepinephrine. Milnacipran is an SNRI approved for treatment of fibromyalgia.

> A related drug, atomoxetine, which is a selective norepinephrine reuptake inhibitor, is used to treat attention-deficit/hyperactivity disorder (ADHD).

HETEROCYCLICS/TCAs

> The precise mechanism of action of the tricyclic drugs is unknown. These drugs block the reuptake of biogenic amines, including norepinephrine and serotonin.

These drugs were the mainstay in the treatment of depression until the SSRIs became available. Most of the drugs in this class are really tricyclics, based on their chemical structure of a three-ring core (Figure 18–1). A couple of other useful antidepressants do not have the three-ring core but otherwise are similar in action

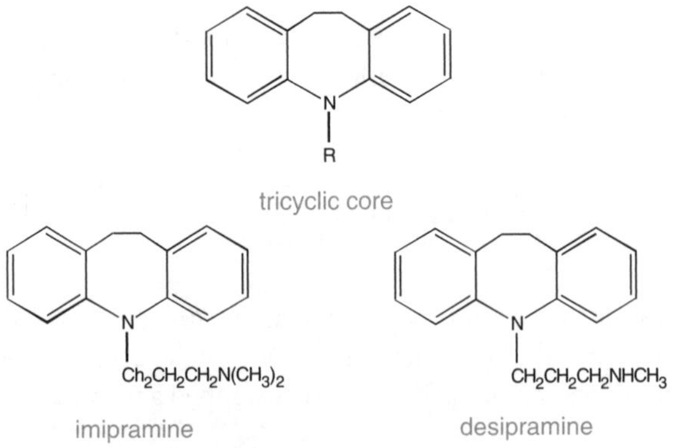

tricyclic core

imipramine   desipramine

FIGURE 18–1 This figure shows the main structure of the tricyclic antidepressants and two examples of drugs in this class. The three rings are obvious.

and side effects to the tricyclic compounds. Therefore, they should all be learned together. The drugs are equally efficacious but vary in potency. In addition, some patients will respond to one drug in this class and not to another one.

Tricyclics have little effect in normal (nondepressed) people. As with most of the antidepressants, 2-3 weeks of dosing with the tricyclics are required before an effect on depression is detectable.

> Heterocyclic antidepressants are
> **1.** Potent muscarinic cholinergic antagonists
> **2.** Weak α_1 antagonists
> **3.** Weak H_1 antagonists
> These actions account for the major side effects of these drugs.

If you can remember these three actions of the heterocyclic antidepressants, then you can also list most of the significant side effects based on your knowledge of autonomic pharmacology (see Chapter 8). The cholinergic blocking effect produces dry mouth, constipation, urinary retention, blurred vision, and so on. The α-blocking effect produces orthostatic hypotension, and the H_1-antagonism produces sedation. Tolerance to the anticholinergic effects does occur.

In overdose, these drugs can produce serious, life-threatening cardiac arrhythmias, delirium, and psychosis.

MONOAMINE OXIDASE (MAO) INHIBITORS

> MAO inhibitors increase levels of norepinephrine, serotonin, and dopamine by inhibiting their degradation.

Although rarely used anymore, MAO inhibitors are antidepressants. Because much is known about these drugs, they still appear in examinations.

Monoamine oxidase is a mitochondrial enzyme that exists in two major forms, A and B. Its major role is to oxidize monoamines, including norepinephrine, serotonin, and dopamine. Blocking this degradative enzyme slows the removal of these transmitters.

Isocarboxazid, phenelzine, and tranylcypromine are irreversible, nonselective inhibitors of MAO-A and MAO-B. However, research suggests that the antidepressant effect of these drugs is due to inhibition of MAO-A.

The potential toxicities of the MAO inhibitors restrict their use.

> MAO inhibitors can cause a *fatal* hypertensive crisis.

Patients who take MAO inhibitors should not take SSRIs or eat foods rich in tyramine or other biologically active amines. These foods include cheese, beer, and red wine. Normally tyramine and other amines are rapidly inactivated by MAO in the gut. Individuals who are taking MAO inhibitors are unable to inactivate the tyramine. The tyramine causes release of norepinephrine, which can lead to an increase in blood pressure and cardiac arrhythmias.

OTHER ANTIDEPRESSANTS

There are now available a number of agents, each in its own unique class. Here we will lump them together as other antidepressants.

> Bupropion is an effective antidepressant that is also approved for use (in combination with behavioral modification) in smoking-cessation programs.

Bupropion is structurally unrelated to the other antidepressants available in the United States. Its mechanism of action is unknown. Bupropion has very few side effects; in particular, it causes less sexual dysfunction than the SSRIs. There is an increased risk of seizures with higher-than-recommended doses. As with the other antidepressants, the therapeutic effect takes several weeks.

Nefazodone and trazodone are structurally unrelated to SSRIs, heterocyclics, or MAO inhibitors. Trazodone is sedative, but nefazodone less so. Nefazodone inhibits serotonin and norepinephrine reuptake, and antagonizes 5-HT$_2$ and α_1 receptors. The α_1-antagonism should tell you that this drug may cause orthostatic hypotension. As with the other antidepressants, the therapeutic effect takes several weeks.

> Mirtazapine is an effective antidepressant that antagonizes central presynaptic α_2 receptors.

Presynaptic α_2 receptors regulate the release of norepinephrine and serotonin. Activation of the receptor reduces the release of norepinephrine and serotonin, whereas blocking the receptor increases norepinephrine and serotonin release. Thus, mirtazapine, which blocks the central presynaptic α_2 receptors, increases release of norepinephrine and serotonin, resulting in an increase in the levels of both neurotransmitters in the synaptic cleft. This mimics the effects of the reuptake inhibitors.

Mirtazapine also interacts with 5-HT receptors. The net result of these interactions is activation of the 5-HT$_{1A}$ receptor. Therefore, it has been classified as a noradrenergic and specific serotonergic antidepressant.

> Sibutramine is a norepinephrine, 5-HT and dopamine reuptake inhibitor that is used as a weight-loss agent.

Although sibutramine is not an antidepressant, it is included here because of the similarity of its mechanism of action. Sibutramine has its effects on the central nervous system, where it inhibits the reuptake of neurotransmitters. The inhibition of reuptake of 5-HT is thought to enhance satiety; the inhibition of reuptake of norepinephrine is thought to increase metabolic rate.

DRUGS USED IN BIPOLAR DISORDER

The main goal of pharmacological treatment of bipolar disorder is to reduce the frequency and severity of fluctuations in mood.

> LITHIUM, carbamazepine, and valproate are drugs used for the treatment of bipolar disorder.

Lithium is still considered the standard treatment for bipolar disorder. However, the anticonvulsants, carbamazepine, valproate, and lamotrigine are also used (see Chapter 21). How any of these drugs work to reduce mood changes is not known. Second-generation antipsychotic drugs (Chapter 19) are also used for treatment of acute mania and for maintenance treatment of bipolar disorder.

> LITHIUM has a low therapeutic index and the frequency and severity of adverse reactions is directly related to the serum levels.

Frequent measurements of the serum level are routinely carried out during chronic treatment. Lithium use is occasionally associated with hypothyroidism or nephrogenic diabetes insipidus.

19 Antipsychotics or Neuroleptics

Organization of Class
Typical Antipsychotics (First Generation)
Serotonin-Dopamine Antagonists (Second Generation)
Neuroleptic Malignant Syndrome

ORGANIZATION OF CLASS

These drugs have been called neuroleptics, antischizophrenic drugs, antipsychotic drugs, and major tranquilizers. All these terms are synonymous; neuroleptic and antipsychotic are the most common. These drugs are not curative (because they do not eliminate the fundamental thinking disorder), but they often permit the patient to function more normally.

> All of the neuroleptics are
> 1. α-Blockers
> 2. Muscarinic antagonists
> 3. Histamine antagonists
> These actions produce the side effects of the drugs.

If you know which receptors these drugs block, you can predict all of the actions and side effects of these drugs. The antimuscarinic actions produce dry mouth, constipation, urinary retention, blurred vision, and so on. The α-antagonism produces orthostatic hypotension, and the H_1-antagonism produces sedation.

These drugs were organized according to their chemical structure. I do not recommend this method unless you have decided to memorize all of the structures. I recommend dividing these drugs into two groups: the older, so-called typical antipsychotics and the newer atypical drugs. The newer "atypical" drugs are now the drugs of choice for the treatment of schizophrenia, so the term "atypical" is a misnomer. The older drugs are now being called "first generation" and the newer drugs "second generation." This makes much more sense. Name recognition here is sometimes a problem, but notice that most of the typical neuroleptics end in "-azine." A number of the second-generation drugs end in "–peridone."

> All neuroleptics are dopamine blockers (D_2), but the atypical drugs (second generation) also block 5-HT$_{2A}$ receptors.

Typical Neuroleptics (First Generation)	5-HT-DA Antagonists (Second Generation)
acetophenazine	amisulpride
CHLORPROMAZINE	aripiprazole
chlorprothixene	asenapine
fluphenazine	CLOZAPINE
HALOPERIDOL	iloperidone
mesoridazine	loxapine
perphenazine	olanzapine
prochlorperazine	paliperidone
thioridazine	quetiapine
thiothixene	RISPERIDONE
trifluoperazine	sertindole
	ziprasidone

You now know the most fundamental information about the drugs in this group. You need only add a little bit more, depending on how much trivia you want to know.

TYPICAL ANTIPSYCHOTICS (FIRST GENERATION)

All the drugs in this group have equal efficacy; they vary only in potency and side effects.

> **REMINDER:** The typical antipsychotics block dopamine, muscarinic cholinergic, α-adrenergic, and H_1-histaminergic receptors.

The dopamine antagonism is believed to produce the antipsychotic effect. It also produces some endocrinological effects. Remember that dopamine inhibits prolactin release. Thus, an antagonist at the dopamine receptor results in an increase in prolactin release. This in turn leads to lactation. Most of the neuroleptics, *except* thioridazine, have antiemetic effects that are mediated by blocking D_2 receptors of the chemoreceptor trigger zone in the medulla.

> All of these drugs produce extrapyramidal effects, including parkinsonism, akathisia, and tardive dyskinesia.

The extrapyramidal effects of these drugs are presumably caused by blocking of dopamine receptors in the striatum (basal ganglia). Extrapyramidal effects include acute dystonia (spasm of the muscles of the face, tongue, neck, and back), akathisia (motor restlessness), and parkinsonism (rigidity, tremor, and shuffling gait). Because it is irreversible, one of the most worrisome extrapyramidal effects is tardive dyskinesia. Tardive dyskinesia may appear during or after prolonged therapy with any of these drugs. It involves stereotyped involuntary movements, such as lip smacking, jaw movements, and darting of the tongue. Purposeless quick movements of the limbs may also occur.

The more potent drugs produce more extrapyramidal effects. Conversely, the drugs with more anticholinergic potency have fewer extrapyramidal effects (Figure 19–1). Compare this to what we know about Parkinson disease. In Parkinson disease, a loss of dopamine neurons leads to a movement disorder that can be treated with anticholinergics. Here, we are using drugs to block dopamine receptors, which you may predict will lead to parkinsonism (symptoms that are similar to Parkinson disease, but not caused by a loss of neurons). Drugs with anticholinergic actions cause fewer extrapyramidal effects because the dopamine–acetylcholine balance in the motor systems is less affected.

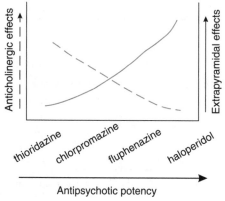

FIGURE 19–1 As the antipsychotics increase in potency for their antipsychotic effect, there is a trend toward a decrease in the anticholinergic side effects (dashed line) and an increase in the incidence of extrapyramidal side effects (solid line).

SEROTONIN-DOPAMINE ANTAGONISTS (SECOND GENERATION)

> Second-generation neuroleptics reduce both the positive and negative symptoms of schizophrenia, while causing a minimum of extrapyramidal side effects.

Although referred to as a serotonin-dopamine antagonist, each agent in this class has a unique combination of receptor affinities. At the very least you should know that these drugs are antagonists at dopamine and 5-HT$_{2A}$ receptors. The affinities for the other receptors determine the side-effect profile. This is the type of information that you can add later. The ability of these drugs to reduce the negative features of psychosis (withdrawal, flat affect, anhedonia, catatonia) and the positive symptoms (hallucinations, delusions, disordered thought, agitation) has led to the use of these drugs in a wide variety of patients.

Clozapine has caused *fatal* agranulocytosis. In patients receiving clozapine, monitoring of the white cell count needs to be done on a regular basis. Agranulocytosis does not appear to be a problem with the newer agents in this class.

> **REMINDER:** The second-generation antipsychotics also block muscarinic, α_1-adrenergic, serotonin, and histamine receptors in addition to dopamine and serotonin receptors.

The side effects you learned for the whole class apply to these drugs as well.

> RISPERIDONE is the drug of choice for new onset schizophrenia.

NEUROLEPTIC MALIGNANT SYNDROME

> Neuroleptic malignant syndrome is a rare, potentially *fatal* neurological side effect of antipsychotic medication.

Many courses do not cover neuroleptic malignant syndrome, but because it is potentially fatal, it is worth a mention here. Neuroleptic malignant syndrome resembles a very severe form of parkinsonism, with catatonia, autonomic instability, and stupor. It may persist for more than a week after administration of the offending drug is stopped. Because mortality is high (10-20%), immediate medical attention is required. This syndrome has occurred with all neuroleptics but is more common with relatively high doses of the more potent agents, especially when administered parenterally.

20 Drugs Used in Parkinson Disease

Organization of Class
Dopamine Replacement Therapy
Dopamine Agonist Therapy
Anticholinergic Therapy

ORGANIZATION OF CLASS

The drugs in this class are arranged by mechanism of action. The groups are quite easy to remember if you remember the pathology of Parkinson disease.

In Parkinson disease there is loss of the dopamine-containing neurons in the substantia nigra (Figure 20–1). These neurons normally project to the caudate putamen (one piece of the basal ganglia) where the dopamine inhibits firing of the cholinergic neurons. These cholinergic neurons form excitatory synapses onto other neurons that project out of the basal ganglia. The result of the loss of dopamine-containing neurons is that the cholinergic neurons are now without their normal inhibition. This is a bit like a car going down a hill without any brakes.

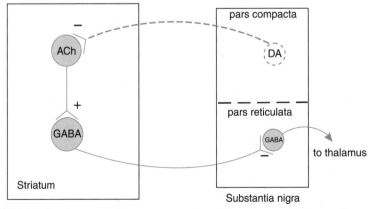

FIGURE 20–1 Diagram of projections into and out of the striatum. In Parkinson disease there is a loss of the dopamine (DA)-containing neurons that project from the substantia nigra to the striatum where they inhibit cholinergic (ACh) neurons (dashed line).

> **THERAPY FOR PARKINSON DISEASE**
> **1.** Dopamine replacement therapy
> **2.** Dopamine agonist therapy
> **3.** Anticholinergic therapy

The goals of therapy are to correct the imbalance of the cholinergic neurons in the striatum. All of the therapeutic approaches to Parkinson disease make sense. Given the loss of dopamine-containing neurons, you could replace the dopamine or give dopamine agonists (to mimic the action of the lost dopamine). Because many of the cholinergic neurons are uninhibited, you could give an anticholinergic drug to try to restore inhibition. If you can remember this much, you are well on your way to a good grasp of this area.

DOPAMINE REPLACEMENT THERAPY

It would be nice if we could just give dopamine itself. However, dopamine does not cross the blood–brain barrier.

> LEVODOPA (L-dopa) is a metabolic precursor of dopamine that crosses the blood-brain barrier (Figure 20–2).

Large doses of levodopa are required because much of the drug is decarboxylated to dopamine in the periphery. All this dopamine floating around peripherally causes side effects.

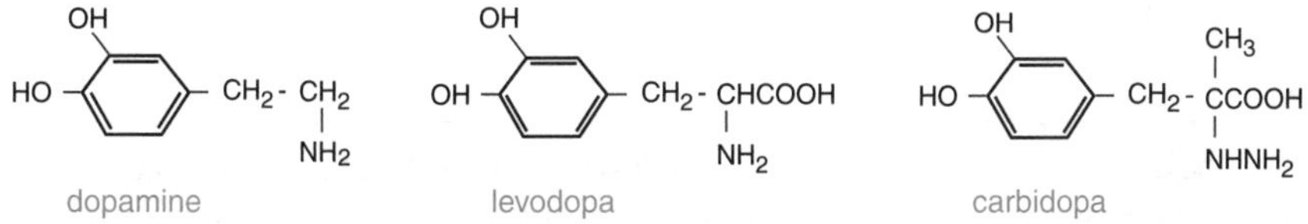

FIGURE 20–2 Structures of dopamine, levodopa, and carbidopa.

> CARBIDOPA is a dopamine decarboxylase inhibitor that does not cross the blood–brain barrier. It reduces the peripheral metabolism of levodopa, thereby increasing the amount of levodopa that reaches the brain.

Carbidopa and levodopa are used today in combination. This is a prime example of a beneficial drug interaction that is logical based on the mechanisms of action of the two drugs. Side effects of levodopa and carbidopa are related to the dopamine that is generated by peripheral decarboxylation.

Tolcapone and entacapone are plasma catechol-o-methyltransferase (COMT) inhibitors that prolong the half-life of levodopa.

> SELEGILINE (also known as deprenyl) is an inhibitor of monoamine oxidase (MAO)-B, the enzyme that metabolizes dopamine in the central nervous system (CNS).

Selegiline is also known as deprenyl and both names appear in books and articles in the medical literature. Inhibition of MAO-B slows the breakdown of dopamine; thus, dopamine remains in the vicinity of its receptors on the cholinergic neurons for a longer period of time. Rasagiline is a newer MAO inhibitor for Parkinson disease.

Amantadine is an antiviral drug effective in the treatment of influenza. It appears to enhance the synthesis, release, or reuptake of dopamine from the surviving nigral neurons, so it can also be used in Parkinson disease.

DOPAMINE AGONIST THERAPY

Dopamine agonists can be used in Parkinson disease because although the dopamine-releasing neurons have disappeared, the postsynaptic dopamine receptors are still present and functional. Administration of dopamine agonists to stimulate these receptors should therefore restore the balance of inhibition and excitation in the basal ganglia.

The main role of these drugs is in combination with levodopa and carbidopa in early Parkinson disease. Dopamine agonists used in the treatment of Parkinson disease include bromocriptine, pergolide, pramipexole, ropinirole, and rotigotine. Pramipexole, ropinirole, and rotigotine are nonergot chemicals, while bromocriptine and pergolide are ergotamine derivatives. The actions and side effects of these drugs are similar to those of levodopa. Activation of dopamine receptors in the pituitary gland inhibits prolactin release. This reduction in prolactin can alter reproductive function.

ANTICHOLINERGIC THERAPY

Anticholinergic agents are less commonly used than the drugs previously reviewed, but they are always taught in pharmacology courses. They reduce the activity of the uninhibited cholinergic neurons in the basal ganglia. These drugs are muscarinic antagonists and differ only in potency. You should be able to list the side effects of muscarinic antagonists from your study of autonomic pharmacology (see Chapter 8). Therefore, there is really little that is new here. However, the drug names are quite awkward and not easily recognizable as antimuscarinic agents.

> Trihexyphenidyl, benztropine, and biperiden are muscarinic antagonists used in Parkinson disease.

Side effects of these drugs include dry mouth, constipation, urinary retention, and confusion. The dopamine agonists and anticholinergics are good candidates for your drug name recognition list.

Antiepileptic Drugs

Organization of Class
Important Details About the Most Important Drugs
Other Drugs to Consider

ORGANIZATION OF CLASS

This class of drugs does not lend itself to the type of organization used in many other chapters. Here we need to consider the disease to be treated.

Epilepsy is a chronic disorder characterized by recurrent episodes in which the brain is subject to abnormal excessive discharges (seizures) synchronized throughout a population of neurons. The seizures themselves have been classified to assist with demographics and treatment. The accompanying table provides a simplified seizure classification scheme.

Seizure Type	Clinical Manifestations
I. Partial (focal, local)	
A. Partial simple	Focal motor, sensory, or speech disturbance. No impairment of consciousness.
B. Partial complex	Dreamy state with automatisms. Impaired consciousness.
C. Partial seizures with secondary generalization	
II. Generalized seizures	
A. Generalized convulsive (tonic-clonic, grand mal)	Loss of consciousness, falling, rigid extension of trunk and limbs. Rhythmic contractions of arms and legs.
B. Generalized nonconvulsive (absence, petit mal)	Impaired consciousness with staring and eye blinks.

Notice that some of these seizures do not involve muscle jerking or convulsions. In particular, absence seizures are called nonconvulsive. Technically, this would make the name *anticonvulsants* inaccurate, but it is often used to designate this class of drugs.

Now that we have defined the types of seizures we want to control, we can start examining the drugs. To simplify this organization, let's consider which drugs are used for which types of seizures. There is not 100% agreement on which is the best drug in each category, so do not be bothered by discrepancies between textbooks.

Seizure Type	Drugs of Choice
Generalized convulsive	VALPROATE
	lamotrigine
	levetiracetam
Partial, including simple, complex and secondarily generalized	CARBAMAZEPINE
	lamotrigine
	oxcarbazepine
	levetiracetam
Generalized nonconvulsive	ETHOSUXIMIDE
	VALPROATE

We have covered the drugs of choice for all of the major types of seizures using only six drugs. In addition to these drugs, you should be aware that there are others available.

IMPORTANT DETAILS ABOUT THE MOST IMPORTANT DRUGS

VALPROATE is associated with elevated liver enzymes, nausea and vomiting, and weight gain. It can also produce a tremor.

Valproate may produce *fatal* hepatic failure. This is most common in children under the age of 2 years who are taking more than one antiepileptic drug. The hepatotoxicity is not dose related; it is considered to be an idiosyncratic reaction.

CARBAMAZEPINE causes autoinduction of its own metabolism.

Carbamazepine is metabolized by the liver and over a period of several weeks induces the enzymes that metabolize it. Therefore, an initially adequate dose gradually produces lower and lower plasma levels as the liver increases the metabolism (shortening the half-life). Carbamazepine has been associated with granulocyte suppression and aplastic anemia.

Oxcarbazepine is chemically similar to carbamazepine, but does not induce liver enzymes to the sane extent.

ETHOSUXIMIDE is the *drug of choice* for absence seizures. It is associated with stomachaches, vomiting, and hiccups.

Ethosuximide is thought to act by blocking calcium channels in the thalamus.

Lamotrigine is a well tolerated antiepileptic agent that is as effective as carbamazepine. It has also been reported to improve depression in some patients with epilepsy.

Levetiracetam binds to a synaptic vesicle protein called SV2A, but the relevance of this for its anticonvulsant activity is not yet known.

OTHER DRUGS TO CONSIDER

Phenytoin used to be widely used in the treatment of epilepsy, but has been largely replaced in the United States with the newer drugs. However, much is known about the pharmacology of phenytoin, particularly the pharmacokinetics.

> PHENYTOIN has zero-order kinetics.

Review the section on zero-order kinetics in Chapter 4 if this does not ring a loud bell for you. The fact that phenytoin has zero-order kinetics is particularly important because phenytoin turns into a zero-order drug right in the therapeutic range (Figure 21–1).

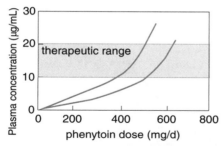

FIGURE 21–1 Plasma concentrations at steady state as a function of dose are shown for two different people. Notice that as the dose of phenytoin increases, the plasma concentration does not follow in a linear fashion. Instead, the curve becomes steeper. That is where phenytoin is switching to zero-order kinetics. This transition occurs at different points for different people.

> PHENYTOIN causes ataxia and nystagmus at high doses. It has been associated with hirsutism, coarsening of facial features, and gingival hyperplasia.

Phenytoin is thought to act by blocking the sodium channel in the inactivated state. If you are interested, you can learn additional details about its side effects and actions

We are getting lower down on the trivia list. If you have learned most of the material we have reviewed so far, please continue. If you have had any trouble with the preceding material, you may wish to wait and add the following details during your second or third pass through.

There are several relatively new drugs that are effective antiepileptic agents in some patients. These include felbamate (has caused aplastic anemia), gabapentin (also used for pain control), fosphenytoin (soluble prodrug for phenytoin), lacosamide, topiramate, tiagabine, and zonisamide.

> Clonazepam is an alternative drug for the treatment of generalized nonconvulsive seizures. It is a benzodiazepine and tolerance develops to its antiepileptic effects.

Chapter 17, on anxiolytics and hypnotics, contains additional features about the benzodiazepines. Use what you learned there and apply it here. Again, do not memorize this drug in isolation.

You should also take a few minutes to review the drugs used in the treatment of status epilepticus before moving on.

Narcotics (Opiates)

Organization of Class
Actions of Morphine and the Other Agonists
Distinguishing Features of Some Agonists
Opioid Antagonists
Opioid Agonist-Antagonists

ORGANIZATION OF CLASS

The word *narcotics* (or *opiates*) refers to drugs that act on specific receptors in the central nervous system (CNS) to reduce perception of pain. In general they do not eliminate pain, but the patient is not as bothered by the pain. They act on three major classes of receptors in the CNS, called opioid receptors and designated mu (μ), kappa (κ), and delta (δ). Most of the actions of the narcotic analgesics are mediated by the μ receptor. Some actions are mediated through the κ and δ receptors.

Divide the narcotics into four groups:
1. Agonists; use morphine as the prototype
2. Weak agonist/reuptake inhibitors
3. Mixed agonist-antagonists
4. Antagonists

A partial listing of drugs in this class is included in the following table.

Agonists	Weak Agonists/ Reuptake Inhibitors	Mixed Agonist-Antagonists	Antagonists
alfentanil	tapentadol	PENTAZOCINE	NALOXONE
CODEINE	tramadol	buprenorphine	NALTREXONE
dihydrocodeine		butorphanol	nalmefene
FENTANYL		dezocine	alvimopan
HEROIN		nalbuphine	

(Continued)

Agonists	Weak Agonists/ Reuptake Inhibitors	Mixed Agonist-Antagonists	Antagonists
hydrocodone			methylnaltrexone
hydromorphone			
levorphanol			
MEPERIDINE			
METHADONE			
MORPHINE			
oxycodone			
oxymorphone			
propoxyphene			
sufentanil			

The most important drug names in this class are in capital letters in the table. Notice that there are many more agonists than antagonists and that there is only one important mixed agonist-antagonist.

> Remember the names of the antagonists (NALOXONE and NALTREXONE) and the most important mixed agonist-antagonist (PENTAZOCINE). Everything else is an agonist.

Of course, that statement was somewhat simplified. Use morphine as the prototype drug in this class. The other agonists have the same general properties. They vary in things like potency and duration of action.

ACTIONS OF MORPHINE AND THE OTHER AGONISTS

> Morphine causes
> 1. Analgesia
> 2. Respiratory depression
> 3. Spasm of smooth muscle of the gastrointestinal (GI) and genitourinary (GU) tracts, including the biliary tract
> 4. Pinpoint pupils

Morphine has actions in many organ systems. We will consider them one at a time. These actions are sometimes used for therapeutic purposes and sometimes are considered side effects. Therefore, learning the important actions means that you have learned both therapeutic uses and adverse effects at one time.

CNS In most people morphine produces drowsiness and sedation in addition to the reduction in awareness of pain. Initial doses of morphine often cause nausea, more often in ambulatory patients than in those who are bedridden. This effect is due to direct stimulation of the chemoreceptor trigger zone in the medulla oblongata and to an increase in vestibular sensitivity.

Morphine is an effective cough suppressant because it has a direct effect in the medulla. Morphine is not used for this purpose, but codeine (another agonist) is frequently prescribed for its cough suppressive action.

EYE Morphine produces pupillary constriction by a direct action in the brain nucleus of the oculomotor nerve (Edinger-Westphal). This is the classic pinpoint pupil that you will hear mentioned in the emergency room.

RESPIRATORY Again, through a direct action on the CNS, morphine causes respiratory depression. All phases of respiratory activity are depressed, including rate and minute volume. The hypoxic drive for breathing is also depressed.

CARDIOVASCULAR (CV) Morphine has essentially no effect on the cardiovascular system at therapeutic doses.

GI Morphine increases the resting tone of the smooth muscle of the entire GI tract. This results in a decrease in the movement of stomach and intestinal contents, which may lead to spasm (pain) and to constipation. Morphine also produces spasm of the smooth muscle of the biliary tract. Tolerance does not develop to the constipating action. Two μ-receptor antagonists that do not cross the blood–brain barrier (alvimopan and methylnaltrexone) can be used to relieve the constipation.

GU Similar to its action on the GI tract, morphine increases the tone and produces spasm of the smooth muscle in the GU tract. This can lead to urinary retention.

> Withdrawal from narcotics in a dependent person consists of autonomic hyperactivity, such as diarrhea, vomiting, chills, fever, tearing, and runny nose. Tremor, abdominal cramps, and pain can be severe.

That was a quick summary of the most important information about morphine's actions. If you are doing well upto this point, then continue and learn some specific details of some of the agonists. If you have some trouble with the preceding details, review the next section on another pass through the material.

DISTINGUISHING FEATURES OF SOME AGONISTS

> CODEINE is used for suppressing cough and for pain. It is much less potent than morphine.

> HEROIN is more lipid soluble than morphine and, therefore, rapidly crosses the blood–brain barrier. It is hydrolyzed to morphine in the brain; thus it is a prodrug.

> MEPERIDINE is less potent than morphine and less spasmogenic. It has no cough suppressive ability.

Here are a few more things that you may need to know. Meperidine is also used in obstetrics. Unlike morphine, meperidine produces no more respiratory depression in the fetus than in the mother.

Two relatives of meperidine (diphenoxylate and loperamide) have gained acceptance for the treatment of diarrhea. Neither is well absorbed after oral administration, so their action remains in the GI tract.

> FENTANYL is 80 times more potent then morphine but has a short duration of action. It is used by anesthesiologists.

> METHADONE is a highly effective analgesic after oral administration and has a much longer duration of action than morphine.

Methadone is used in the treatment of patients addicted to narcotics. This use appears counterintuitive to some students. The knee jerk impulse is to think of treating addicts with an antagonist. That approach, however, would put them into immediate and frightening withdrawal. The idea behind methadone treatment is to replace the addict's heroin with an orally active agonist that has a long duration of action. This reduces the drug craving and prevents the symptoms of withdrawal. Do not be tempted to think of methadone as an antagonist.

> The weak agonist/reuptake inhibitors are μ-agonists and norepinephrine (and serotonin) reuptake inhibitors.

Before we leave the agonists, you should be aware that the opiates are often used in combination with the nonopiate analgesics (aspirin and acetaminophen). Because these different classes of drugs affect pain pathways by different mechanisms, the combinations have proven to be effective in producing analgesia with fewer side effects.

OPIOID ANTAGONISTS

> Opioid antagonists have no effect when administered alone. When given after a dose of agonist, they promptly reverse all of the actions of the agonist.

This is basically the definition of an antagonist from general principles.

> NALOXONE is the *drug of choice* for narcotic overdose.

OPIOID AGONIST-ANTAGONISTS

The concept of a mixed agonist-antagonist is confusing to many students. These drugs appear to be agonists at the κ receptor, which gives them analgesic activity. They are also antagonists at the μ receptor. This leads to their classification as mixed agonist-antagonists.

> PENTAZOCINE produces effects that are qualitatively similar to morphine.

> PENTAZOCINE causes acute withdrawal in patients who have received regular doses of morphine or other agonists.

General Anesthetics

Organization of Class
Uptake and Distribution of Inhalational Anesthetics
Elimination of Inhalational Anesthetics
Potency of General Anesthetics
Specific Gases and Volatile Liquids
Specific Intravenous Agents

ORGANIZATION OF CLASS

The state of general anesthesia is a drug-induced absence of perception of all sensations. Depths of anesthesia appropriate for surgical procedures can be achieved with a wide variety of drugs. General anesthetics are administered primarily by inhalation and intravenous (IV) injection. These routes of administration allow control of the dosage and time course of action.

For these drugs, understanding the principles of uptake, distribution, and elimination are the major focus, particularly for the inhaled anesthetics. The mechanism of action of most of the anesthetics is unknown. You should be able to recognize the names of the general anesthetics and know a few specific facts about these drugs (Figure 23–1).

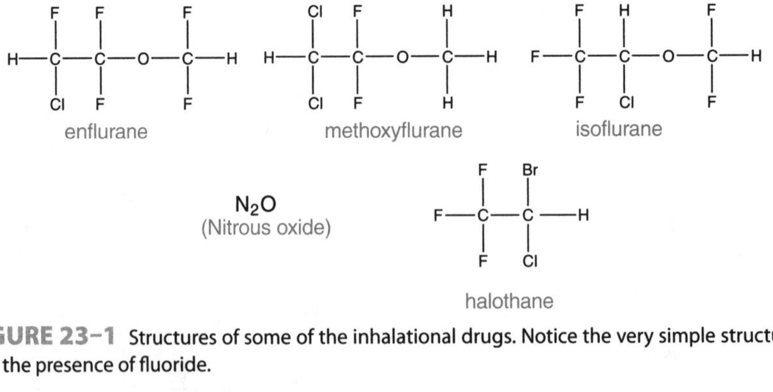

FIGURE 23–1 Structures of some of the inhalational drugs. Notice the very simple structures and the presence of fluoride.

Inhaled Drugs	IV Drugs
desflurane	PROPOFOL
ENFLURANE	THIOPENTAL
HALOTHANE	etomidate
ISOFLURANE	ketamine
NITROUS OXIDE	
methoxyflurane	
sevoflurane	

UPTAKE AND DISTRIBUTION OF INHALATIONAL ANESTHETICS

The tension of a gas in a mixture is proportional to its concentration. Therefore, the terms *tension* and *concentration* are often used interchangeably. The term *partial pressure* is also used interchangeably with tension.

> When a constant tension (concentration) of anesthetic gas is inhaled, the tension (concentration) in arterial blood approaches that of the agent in the inspired mixture. The tension (concentration) in the brain is always approaching the tension (concentration) in arterial blood.

The level of general anesthesia is dependent on the concentration of anesthetic in the brain.

> The solubility of an agent is expressed as the blood:gas partition coefficient.

The blood:gas partition coefficient represents the ratio of anesthetic concentration in blood to the concentration in the gas phase. The blood:gas coefficient is high for very soluble agents and low for relatively insoluble anesthetics such as nitrous oxide.

> The more soluble an anesthetic is in blood, the more of it must be dissolved in blood to raise its partial pressure in the blood.

The potential reservoir for relatively soluble gases is large and will be filled more slowly. Therefore, for soluble gases the rate at which the tension (partial pressure) in the arterial blood approaches the inspired partial pressure is slow. Also, the rate at which the brain partial pressure approaches the arterial partial pressure is slow. The opposite is true for more insoluble anesthetics.

> The speed of onset of anesthesia is inversely related to the solubility of the gas in blood:
> More soluble (high blood:gas partition coefficient) = slower onset
> Less soluble (low blood:gas partition coefficient) = faster onset

Onset of anesthesia is also related to pulmonary ventilation, rate of pulmonary blood flow, tissue blood flow, and solubility of the gas in the tissues.

ELIMINATION OF INHALATIONAL ANESTHETICS

> Elimination of anesthetics is influenced by pulmonary ventilation, blood flow, and solubility of the gas.

The major factors that affect the rate of elimination of the anesthetics are the same factors that are important in the uptake phase. This makes these principles easy to remember.

Most of the inhaled anesthetics are eliminated unchanged in the exhaled gas. A small percentage of the anesthetics are metabolized in the liver. It has been suggested that the production of a toxic metabolite may be responsible for most of the hepatic and renal toxicities observed with these agents. One example of this is methoxyflurane. It has been associated with renal failure as a result of the toxic amounts of fluoride ions that are produced when the drug is metabolized. More details about this process are available in your pharmacology textbook.

POTENCY OF GENERAL ANESTHETICS

Anesthesiologists have accepted a measure of potency for the inhalational anesthetics known as the minimum alveolar concentration (MAC).

> Minimum alveolar concentration (MAC) is defined as the alveolar concentration at one atmosphere that produces immobility in 50% of patients exposed to a painful stimulus.

The MAC is usually expressed as the percentage of gas in the mixture required to achieve immobility in 50% of patients exposed to a painful stimulus. The alveolar concentration is used for this definition because the concentration in the lung can be easily and accurately measured. The real concentration that we would want to know is the brain concentration. It is not so easy to measure brain levels, but we know that brain levels are directly correlated to alveolar levels. So, the MAC is a good approximation of brain levels.

SPECIFIC GASES AND VOLATILE LIQUIDS

Each of these drugs has a whole range of effects on the lungs, heart, and circulation. It is probably advisable to read through a detailed description of these effects and pick out some trends to memorize.

> NITROUS OXIDE is a relatively insoluble gas, with a MAC of about 105%, that has little effect on blood pressure or respiration. It does produce analgesia.

The low solubility means that onset of anesthesia with nitrous oxide is very fast. The MAC indicates that nitrous oxide has very low potency—so low in fact, that more than 100% of the inspired gas needs to be nitrous oxide to produce immobility in 50% of patients exposed to a painful stimulus. That is why nitrous oxide is used in combination with other agents.

SPECIFIC INTRAVENOUS AGENTS

Some barbiturates (thiopental and methohexital) and benzodiazepines (midazolam) are used for anesthesia, particularly during induction. They are covered in Chapter 17. Thus, for our purposes here, it is just a matter of adding what you already know about barbiturates and benzodiazepines to these names and associating them with anesthesia. These drugs do not produce analgesia.

The majority of IV drugs used to induce anesthesia are slowly metabolized and excreted, and depend on redistribution to terminate their pharmacological effects.

> PROPOFOL and etomidate are two drugs used intravenously to produce general anesthesia.

On your first pass, you should recognize these names and know that they are general anesthetics. On the second pass, you should try to add some details about analgesia and cardiovascular effects.

Local Anesthetics

Organization of Class
Mechanism of Action
Special Features about Individual Agents

ORGANIZATION OF CLASS

These drugs are applied locally and block nerve conduction. Nerve fibers are not affected equally. Loss of sympathetic function occurs first, followed by loss of pinprick sensation and temperature, and, lastly, motor function. The effect of local anesthetics is reversible: their use is followed by complete recovery of nerve function with no evidence of structural damage.

All the local anesthetics consist of a hydrophilic amino group linked through a connecting group of variable length to a lipophilic aromatic portion (benzene ring, Figure 24–1). In the intermediate chain, there is either an ester linkage or an amide linkage.

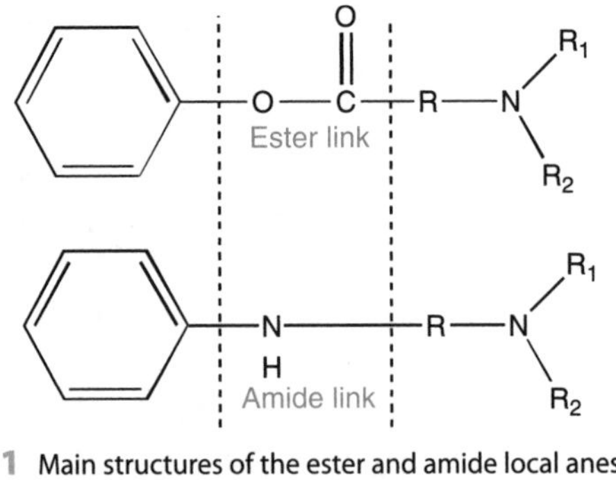

FIGURE 24–1 Main structures of the ester and amide local anesthetics.

The commonly used local anesthetics can be classified as esters or amides based on the linkage in this intermediate chain. It is not as important to know which drugs are esters and which are amides, as it is to know that there is a difference. The amide local anesthetics are chemically stable in vivo, whereas the esters are rapidly hydrolyzed by plasma cholinesterase. One interesting but trivial fact is that metabolism of the ester local anesthetics leads to formation of para-aminobenzoic acid (PABA), which is thought to be allergenic.

ESTERS	AMIDES
COCAINE	LIDOCAINE
PROCAINE	bupivacaine
benzocaine	etidocaine
chlorprocaine	mepivacaine
tetracaine	prilocaine
	ropivacaine
	articaine
	levobupivacaine

The "-caine" ending on each of these drug names tells you that they are local anesthetics.

> Adverse effects of the local anesthetics result from systemic absorption of toxic amounts of the drugs.

Death can occur from respiratory failure secondary to medullary depression or from hypotension and cardiovascular collapse.

MECHANISM OF ACTION

> Local anesthetics block the sodium channel in the nerve membrane.

Application of a local anesthetic inhibits the inward movement of Na^+ ions. This results in elevation of the threshold for electrical excitation, reduction in the rate of rise of the action potential, and slowing of the propagation of the impulse. At high enough concentrations, the local anesthetics completely block conduction of impulses down the nerve.

For those of you interested in this area, there is a fascinating story relating pH to ionization of the local anesthetics to drug action. For details, see your textbook.

SPECIAL FEATURES ABOUT INDIVIDUAL AGENTS

> LIDOCAINE is a local anesthetic used intravenously in the treatment of cardiac arrhythmias.

> COCAINE is better known as a drug of abuse, but it is also an effective local anesthetic.

PART V Chemotherapeutic Agents

CHAPTER 25:   Introduction to Chemotherapy   131

CHAPTER 26:   Inhibitors of Cell Wall Synthesis   136

CHAPTER 27:   Protein Synthesis Inhibitors   142

CHAPTER 28:   Folate Antagonists   147

CHAPTER 29:   Quinolones and Urinary Tract Antiseptics   149

CHAPTER 30:   Drugs Used in Tuberculosis and Leprosy   151

CHAPTER 31:   Antifungal Drugs   155

CHAPTER 32:   Anthelmintic Drugs   159

CHAPTER 33:   Antiviral Drugs   162

CHAPTER 34:   Antiprotozoal Drugs   166

CHAPTER 35:   Anticancer Drugs   170

Introduction to Chemotherapy

Approach to the Antimicrobials
General Principles of Therapy
Definitions
Important Concepts to Understand
Classification of Antimicrobials

APPROACH TO THE ANTIMICROBIALS

Students often have difficulty with the antibiotics, not because of any difficult concepts, but because of the large number of drugs in this class. It can also be overwhelming to try to memorize the organisms that are sensitive to each drug.

Try this approach. First, make absolutely sure that you understand the general principles of therapy and some definitions. We'll go over these in this chapter.

Second, be aware of the classes of antibiotics and the mechanism of action for the class. Note any features that are common to all drugs in the class.

Third, learn the particular adverse effects or special features of administration for the drugs in the class. Do any of the drugs cause potentially *fatal* side effects?

Fourth, learn the broad categories of bacterial spectrum and whether any of the drugs in the class are the *drug of choice* for the treatment of a particular organism. For example, are the drugs good against all of the gram-positive bacteria, but none of the gram-negative? It may be useful to quickly review the most common bacteria at this point. Can you say which bacteria are gram positive and which are gram negative? A solid knowledge of this content will really help when you try to learn about antibiotics. Remember that the sensitivity of bacteria to antibiotics changes over time and in different locations.

This looks like a long list of things to learn, but it is really quite manageable. Don't get too bogged down in trying to remember the second-line drugs for treatment of certain organisms or which drug to use in case of allergies, and so on. This can be added later to the base of knowledge that you develop now.

GENERAL PRINCIPLES OF THERAPY

To be a useful antibiotic, a compound should inhibit the growth of bacteria without harming the human host.

This should be self-evident, but it is the basis for understanding most of the mechanisms of action of these drugs. The compound should affect some aspect of bacteria that is not present in mammalian cells. We'll come back to that later.

> The drug should penetrate body tissues in order to reach the bacteria.

This again should be self-evident. Again, this is the basis for knowing whether a drug is orally absorbed and whether it will cross the blood–brain barrier. For example, if the patient has a GI infection, then you would give a drug orally that is not absorbed by the GI tract. The bacteria are thus treated and the patient has few side effects. Likewise, the drugs that are used to treat meningitis are ones that cross the blood–brain barrier. The drug that is extremely effective against *Haemophilus influenzae* does no good for the patient if it cannot reach the organisms.

DEFINITIONS

> *Spectrum*—as in narrow, broad, and extended—is a term used to convey an impression of the range of bacteria that a drug is effective against.

Drugs are designated as narrow spectrum if they are only effective against one class of bacteria. They are designated as broad spectrum if they are effective against a range of bacteria. If a narrow-spectrum agent is modified chemically (as in adding a new side chain), and the new compound is effective against more bacteria than the parent compound, then the new drug is said to have an extended spectrum. This is easy enough.

> Bacteriostatic versus bactericidal—be sure you know the difference.

Textbooks often place a lot of emphasis on whether a drug will arrest the growth and replication of a bacteria (-static) or actually kill the bacteria (-cidal). If a drug is bacteriostatic, the patient's immune system must complete the task of clearing the body of the invaders. However, these terms are relative and not always accurate. Some drugs can kill one type of bug (-cidal) and only arrest the growth of another (-static). So, don't focus too much time on this early on.

IMPORTANT CONCEPTS TO UNDERSTAND

> Resistance of bacteria to an antibiotic can occur by mutation, adaptation, or gene transfer.

The whole area of bacterial resistance has received much attention lately and appropriately so. Many bacteria are becoming resistant to the available drugs. Students need to have some idea of the mechanisms of bacterial resistance.

Bacteria undergo spontaneous mutation at a frequency of about 1 in 10^{16} cells. Mutation may make bacteria resistant to an antibiotic, or it may not.

Adaptation can take several routes. The bacteria may alter the uptake of the drug by changes in their lipopolysaccharide coat. Or they may improve a transport system that removes the drug from the cell. The bacteria may increase metabolism through a pathway that bypasses the effect of the antibiotic.

Gene transfer occurs through plasmids and transposons. Plasmids are extra-chromosomal genetic elements (pieces of RNA or DNA that are not part of chromosomes). These may code for enzymes that inactivate antimicrobials. The plasmids are transferred from bacteria to bacteria by conjugation and transduction.

Transposons are segments of genetic material with insertion sequences. They are incorporated into the genetic makeup of bacteria and can also code for enzymes that inactivate the antimicrobials.

> Adverse effects can be allergic, toxic, idiosyncratic, or related to changes in the normal body flora.

Adverse effects of antibiotics are grouped into general categories. The first three categories (allergic, toxic, and idiosyncratic) apply to all drugs. The last (changes in normal body flora) is unique to antibiotics.

A reminder: Idiosyncratic reactions are reactions that are not related to immune responses or known drug properties. Examples of idiosyncratic reactions include the hemolysis that occurs in glucose-6-phosphate dehydrogenase (G-6-PD)–deficient patients after treatment with sulfonamides, and the peripheral neuropathy that develops after isoniazid administration in genetically slow acetylators.

The phrase "alterations in the normal body flora" usually refers to changes that occur within the GI tract. Normally the gut is host to friendly bacteria that help in the digestion of the food we eat. If an antimicrobial agent is given orally, it may kill these friendly bacteria. Other bacteria that are resistant to the antimicrobial can then overgrow and repopulate the GI tract. This secondary infection is sometimes called a superinfection. The most common example is the overgrowth of *Clostridium difficile*. It produces a toxin that causes a disorder called pseudomembranous colitis. As you read in your textbook, you will probably see comments about the incidence of colitis after use of a particular antibiotic.

> Combinations of antimicrobial agents can take advantage of the mechanisms of action to produce a synergistic effect.

The area of drug combinations is where an understanding of the mechanisms of action of the antimicrobials becomes important. You can combine agents with different sites of action.

Example: combine a protein synthesis inhibitor (these are bacteriostatic; that is, they stop cell growth) with a drug that affects cell wall synthesis (which requires the cell to be dividing to have an action). Does this combination make sense?

This combination does not make sense. The protein synthesis inhibitor will stop cell growth and prevent cell division so that the second drug will have no effect (except possible side effects).

Example: Two drugs both inhibit production of a key metabolic product, but at two different sites in the metabolic pathway. Does this combination make sense?

This combination is useful. The two drugs, trimethoprim and sulfamethoxazole, inhibit the synthesis of folic acid at different steps in the pathway. They, in a sense, help each other out.

Example: The combination of a cell wall synthesis inhibitor and a drug that needs to act intracellularly. Does this combination make sense?

This combination is extremely useful. It describes the combination of penicillins and aminoglycosides. The penicillins alter the cell wall and enhance the penetration of the aminoglycoside.

> Culture and sensitivity testing will determine the MIC for the bacteria.

The best way to determine the proper antimicrobial agent for a patient is to culture and identify the organism. The laboratory can then run a test for sensitivity of the organism to a series of antimicrobials. They can determine the minimum inhibitory concentration (MIC), which is the lowest concentration of the drug that inhibits growth of the organism. The drug to which the organism is most sensitive has the lowest MIC. Culture and sensitivity (C and S) testing is extremely useful in the selection of the best antimicrobial agent to use but it can take several days, depending on the growth rate of the organism.

Now let's look at the specific drugs.

CLASSIFICATION OF ANTIMICROBIALS

Antimicrobial Drug Classes

Inhibitors of Cell Wall Synthesis

β-Lactams

  aztreonam

  carbapenems

  cephalosporins

  penicillins

Others

  bacitracin

daptomycin

  fosfomycin

  vancomycin

(Continued)

Antimicrobial Drug Classes (*Continued*)

Protein Synthesis Inhibitors

    aminoglycosides

    chloramphenicol

    clindamycin

    macrolides (erythromycin)

    mupirocin

    ketolide

    oxazolidinone

    retapamulin

    streptogramin

    tetracyclines

Folate Antagonists

    sulfonamides and trimethoprim

Quinolones and Other Drugs

    quinolones

    urinary tract antiseptics

Notice how your textbook organizes these drugs. Some books focus primarily on structure and others primarily on mechanisms. Don't let this confuse you. Notice also that there are two really big groups of drugs: the cell wall synthesis inhibitors and the protein synthesis inhibitors. This is in part because bacteria have a cell wall, whereas mammalian cells do not. Also, bacteria have different ribosomal units than mammalian cells. Therefore, targeting cell wall or protein synthesis kills the bacteria and not the host.

CHAPTER

26 Inhibitors of Cell Wall Synthesis

General Features
β-Lactams
    Penicillins
    Cephalosporins
    Carbapenems
    Monobactams (Aztreonam)
Other Inhibitors of Cell Wall Synthesis
    Vancomycin
    Bacitracin
    Fosfomycin
    Daptomycin

GENERAL FEATURES

> The penicillins, cephalosporins, vancomycin, imipenem, and aztreonam all work by inhibiting the synthesis of the bacterial cell wall.

You probably guessed this from the title of the chapter. However, this is a really key point. If you can remember this, you are well on your way to learning these drugs.

The final step in the synthesis of the bacterial cell wall is a cross-linking of adjacent peptidoglycan strands by a process called transpeptidation. The penicillins and cephalosporins are structurally similar to the terminal portion of the peptidoglycan strands and can compete for and bind to the enzymes that catalyze transpeptidation and cross-linking. These enzymes are called penicillin-binding proteins (PBPs). Interference with these enzymes results in the formation of a structurally weakened cell wall, oddly shaped bacteria, and ultimately, death.

Now, let's divide the cell wall synthesis inhibitors into two groups based on chemical structure: β-lactams and polypeptides.

β-LACTAMS

> All of the drugs in this group contain a β-lactam ring in their structure.

Normally, we do not worry too much about the structures of drugs, but in this case we make an important exception. These drugs are often referred to as the β-lactam group. This is because they all have a β-lactam ring in their chemical structure, and it is this β-lactam ring that makes them effective antimicrobials.

> Some bacteria inactivate the β-lactam antibiotics by an enzyme that opens the β-lactam ring.

Some bacteria contain an enzyme, called β-lactamase, that can open the β-lactam ring (Figure 26–1). This leads to inactivation of the antibiotic. The most common mode of drug resistance is plasmid transfer of the genetic code for the β-lactamase enzyme. There is a β-lactamase specific for the penicillins—it is called penicillinase—and a β-lactamase specific for the cephalosporins—it is called cephalosporinase. Is this easy enough? Inactivation of these drugs by β-lactamases is a major problem and has been the focus of intense research.

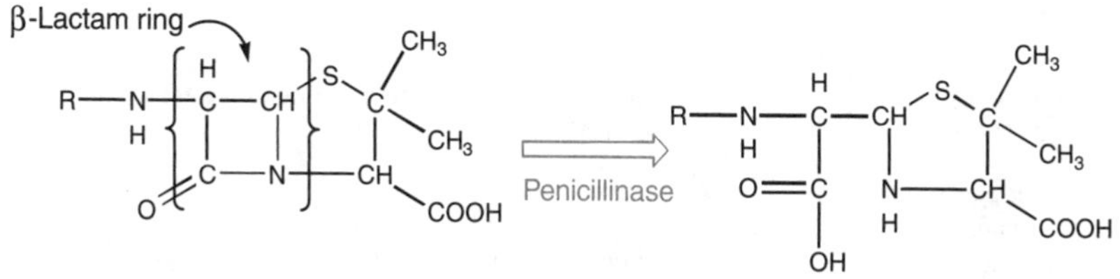

FIGURE 26–1 Here we can see the lactam ring and its opening by penicillinase.

> The inactivation of these drugs by the β-lactamases can be dealt with by two approaches:
> 1. Give a β-lactamase inhibitor at the same time.
> 2. Make chemical modifications in the structure of the drug to make it more resistant to inactivation.

One way to increase the effectiveness of the β-lactam antibiotics is to give a β-lactamase inhibitor at the same time. The most commonly used ones are clavulanic acid and sulbactam. You may also come across tazobactam.

> CLAVULANIC ACID and SULBACTAM are β-lactamase inhibitors that are given together with the β-lactam drugs to increase their effectiveness.

The other approach is to chemically modify the structure of the compounds to make the β-lactam ring more difficult for the enzyme to open.

You now know a lot about the penicillins and cephalosporins and we haven't even listed them yet. See? This is really not too difficult.

PENICILLINS

Most books divide the penicillins into three or four groups. The naturally occurring ones are those that are made by the mold. The rest are chemical modifications of these original penicillins to try to improve the bacterial spectrum and improve resistance to the penicillinase (β-lactamase).

Penicillin Type	Spectrum
Natural PENICILLIN G PENICILLIN V benzathine pen G	Narrow spectrum (gram-positive); penicillinase sensitive
Penicillinase resistant METHICILLIN cloxacillin dicloxacillin nafcillin oxacillin	Narrow spectrum (gram-positive); synthesized to be penicillinase resistant
Aminopenicillins AMOXICILLIN AMPICILLIN	Broad spectrum (some gram-negative activity also); penicillinase sensitive
Extended spectrum azlocillin carbenicillin mezlocillin piperacillin ticarcillin	Active against *Pseudomonas;* relatively ineffective against gram-positive organisms

First of all, notice that the penicillins are easy to identify by the "-cillin" ending. The first group contains the G and V penicillins. The second group contains the three *oxa*cillins. The third group starts with "am-" for amino group. Except for methicillin and nafcillin, the rest are in the last group. Again, this is really not too hard. Keep them categorized and remember the general outline for the spectrum and you'll do just fine.

The oral absorption of the penicillins is poor; however, there are exceptions. If you have time and energy, you can learn the orally active ones. Most of these only cross the blood–brain barrier if it is inflamed. If you have a bit more time, add the ones that can be used in meningitis.

> Penicillins are excreted by tubular secretion that can be blocked by probenecid.

The penicillins are, for the most part, excreted by active tubular secretion. Blocking tubular secretion is a relatively simple way to prolong the action of the drug. Probenecid can be administered along with the penicillins, and it blocks the tubular secretion.

> The most important adverse effect of penicillins as a group is the hypersensitivity reaction. It can be *fatal.*

All penicillins can give rise to allergic reactions. These reactions have been divided into three types: immediate, accelerated, and late. The immediate is the most severe.

The immediate reaction occurs within 20 minutes after parenteral administration and consists of apprehension, itching (pruritus), paresthesia (numbness and tingling), wheezing, choking, fever, edema, and generalized urticaria (hives). It can lead to hypotension, shock, loss of consciousness, and death. The immediate hypersensitivity reaction to penicillin appears to be mediated by IgE antibodies to the minor determinants.

The accelerated reaction appears 1-72 hours after drug administration and it consists mainly of urticaria (hives).

The late reaction is more common with the semisynthetics and appears 72 hours to several weeks after drug administration. It consists mainly of skin rashes.

CEPHALOSPORINS

These drugs are classified into generations. It is impossible to learn all the names (but they almost all begin with "cef" or "ceph"), so focus on the differences between the generations and try to learn three names in each generation. I have listed just the more common ones.

Cephalosporin Type	Spectrum
First generation CEFAZOLIN CEPHALEXIN	Narrow spectrum similar to broad spectrum penicillins; sensitive to β-lactamases
Second generation CEFACLOR CEFAMANDOLE CEFOXITIN	Increased activity toward gram-negative organisms; increased stability
Third generation CEFOTAXIME CEFTAZIDIME CEFTRIAXONE	Even broader in spectrum and more resistant to β-lactamases
Fourth generation cefepime cefpirome	Gram-positive and gram-negative activity, especially against *Pseudomonas aeruginosa;* includes gram-negative organisms with multiple-drug resistance patterns

Believe it or not, this is most of what you need to know. Add a few facts about absorption, distribution, and elimination and you'll be doing great.

Some of these drugs can be given orally (such as cephalexin and cefaclor). You can learn these if you want to try.

The third-generation cephalosporins are used extensively in the treatment and prophylaxis of infections in hospitalized patients. The fourth-generation drugs are being designed to target organisms with multiple-drug resistance.

These drugs are relatively nontoxic. Here are a few facts to consider learning.

1. There is some cross-allergy with penicillins.
2. Some cephalosporins have anti–vitamin K effects (bleeding).
3. Some cephalosporins can cause a disulfiram-like reaction because they block alcohol oxidation, causing acetaldehyde to accumulate.

There is a drug related to the cephalosporins, loracarbef, which is only mentioned here because of the quite different name. You should learn its name with the other cephalosporins, even though technically it is in a different class (the carbacephems).

CARBAPENEMS

This class of β-lactam antibiotics contains imipenem, doripenem, ertapenem, and meropenem. All are administered intravenously.

> IMIPENEM with CILASTATIN is a broad spectrum β-lactam antibiotic.

Imipenem is the antibiotic. It is hydrolyzed by a renal dipeptidase on the luminal brush border of proximal tubular epithelium (that is, in the kidney) to a somewhat toxic metabolite that is inactive as an antimicrobial. Cilastatin inhibits the renal dipeptidase. Therefore, the two compounds are always administered together. Meropenem is more stable to the renal peptidase and does not need the co-administration of cilastin. Note the common "penem" ending of each name.

MONOBACTAMS (AZTREONAM)

The term *monobactam* refers to the chemical structure of this new class of β-lactams. The only one currently available is aztreonam.

> AZTREONAM is an excellent drug for aerobic gram-negative bacteria, including *Pseudomonas*, but it is ineffective against gram-positive organisms.

Aztreonam is an example of a narrow-spectrum drug and is highly resistant to the action of the β-lactamases. It has an unusual spectrum, especially compared to the other β-lactams, so it is a good idea to file this one away in your memory bank.

OTHER INHIBITORS OF CELL WALL SYNTHESIS

These last few drugs are inhibitors of cell wall synthesis, but are not β-lactam compounds.

VANCOMYCIN

Vancomycin, teicoplanin, and telavancin are glycopeptides that inhibit cell wall synthesis by preventing polymerization of the linear peptidoglycans.

> VANCOMYCIN is only effective against the gram-positive organisms. It is very poorly absorbed orally.

Vancomycin can cause a dose-related ototoxicity that produces tinnitus (ringing), high-tone deafness, hearing loss, and possible deafness. This is serious enough to commit to memory.

BACITRACIN

> Bacitracin is a mixture of polypeptides that inhibit cell wall synthesis. It is used topically.

Bacitracin binds to a lipid carrier that transports cell wall precursors to the growing cell wall. Therefore, it can be classified as a cell wall synthesis inhibitor. Because bacitracin has serious nephrotoxicity, it is only used topically.

FOSFOMYCIN

Fosfomycin inhbits one of the first steps in the synthesis of peptidoglycan (ie, the cell wall) by inhibiting the enzyme enolpyruvyl transferase. It is used for the treatment of uncomplicated urinary tract infections.

DAPTOMYCIN

Daptomycin is a lipopeptide antibiotic with a spectrum of activity similar to vancomycin. It binds to the membrane of the bacteria and causes a depolarization of the bacteria. This loss of membrane potential results in bacterial death. So, it is not really an inhibitor of cell wall synthesis, but function.

27 Protein Synthesis Inhibitors

General Features
Aminoglycosides
Tetracyclines
Macrolides
Streptogramins and oxazolidinones
Chloramphenicol
Clindamycin

GENERAL FEATURES

Protein synthesis machinery, including ribosomes, is somewhat different in bacteria compared to mammalian cells. This accounts for the selectivity of this group of drugs for bacteria. Some textbooks and instructors make a point of having students know which ribosomal subunit a class of drugs binds to. However, this is not of primary importance. If you already know it, try not to forget it. If you are struggling with the antimicrobials at this point, save this fact for later. These drugs require binding to an intracellular protein (ribosomal subunit). Therefore, the drugs need to gain entry into the cell. A major route of resistance for the bacteria is to block the movement of the drugs into the cell.

Classes of protein synthesis inhibitors include:

- Aminoglycosides (bactericidal)
- Tetracyclines
- Macrolides (for example, erythromycin)
- Ketolides
- Streptogramins
- Oxazolidinones
- Chloramphenicol
- Clindamycin

These class names are related to the chemical structure of the compounds in each group, but don't worry too much about remembering the class name. It is more important to know the individual drug names here.

AMINOGLYCOSIDES

GENTAMICIN
TOBRAMYCIN
amikacin
kanamycin
neomycin
netilmicin
streptomycin

Notice that the names of these drugs all end in "-mycin" or "-micin," except amikacin. However, the drug companies have thrown you a curve ball here, because the drug clindamycin and all the macrolides (erythromycin, clarithromycin, etc.) also end in "-mycin." So take a moment to compare the list of names here with the one included later in the chapter. Be sure that you can recognize which class a particular name belongs to.

The aminoglycosides are broad-spectrum antimicrobials. However, anaerobic bacteria are generally resistant to them.

Some bacteria use an oxygen-dependent transport system to bring the amino-glycosides into the cell. The anaerobes (with non–oxygen-based metabolism) do not have this system. Therefore, they are generally resistant to the aminoglycosides.

Aminoglycosides are poorly absorbed from the GI tract.

Most aminoglycosides must be administered parenterally. They are highly polar compounds and are relatively insoluble in fat. They do not readily penetrate most cells without help from penicillins or a transport system.

Recall the synergism between penicillins and aminoglycosides that was mentioned in the introduction to chemotherapy (see Chapter 25). The penicillins cause cell wall abnormalities that allow the aminoglycosides to gain entry into the bacteria.

Aminoglycosides have ototoxicity, nephrotoxicity, and neuromuscular toxicity.

The margin of safety with these drugs is small. This means that the toxic concentration is only slightly higher than the therapeutic concentration.

The ototoxicity can be both cochlear (auditory) and vestibular. The symptoms include tinnitus (ringing), deafness, vertigo or unsteadiness of gait, and high-frequency hearing loss. The cochlear toxicity results from selective destruction of the outer hair cells in the organ of Corti.

The nephrotoxicity is related to the rapid uptake of the drug by proximal tubular cells. The proximal tubular cells are then killed. Acute nephrotoxicity is reversible.

The neurotoxicity is caused by the blockade of presynaptic release of acetylcholine at the neuromuscular junction. There is also some postsynaptic blockade as well. This leads to weakness and can lead to respiratory depression.

TETRACYCLINES

TETRACYCLINE
chlortetracycline
demeclocycline
DOXYCYCLINE
minocycline
oxytetracycline

These drug names are easy to recognize, because they all end in "-cycline." Similar to the aminoglycosides, the tetracyclines accumulate in the cytoplasm by an energy-dependent transport system. This transport system is not present in mammalian cells. Resistance to tetracyclines occurs when bacteria mutate in a way that makes them unable to accumulate the drug.

> Tetracyclines are broad-spectrum antibiotics.

Tetracyclines are useful in the treatment of gram-positive and gram-negative facultative organisms and anaerobes.

> Tetracyclines have also found use in rickettsial diseases (Rocky Mountain spotted fever), chlamydial diseases, cholera, Lyme disease (spirochetes), and in mycoplasma pneumonia.

Notice that tetracyclines are useful in the treatment of some oddball diseases, particularly the rickettsiae and spirochetes.

> Food impairs the absorption of the tetracyclines.

Except for doxycycline and minocycline, food impairs the absorption of the tetracyclines. The tetracyclines form insoluble chelates with calcium, magnesium, and other metals. The use of antacids when taking tetracyclines is therefore not advised.

> Tetracyclines are associated with staining of the teeth, retardation of bone growth, and photosensitivity.

The major side effects of the tetracyclines are related to their incorporation into teeth and bone. They cause the teeth to be discolored and can retard bone growth. For these reasons, they are not recommended for use in children or pregnant women. There is an increased incidence of an abnormal sunburn reaction in people taking tetracyclines.

Glycylcyclines are derivatives of the tetracyclines and they also work by inhibiting protein synthesis. Tigecycline is the first drug available in this class.

MACROLIDES

ERYTHROMYCIN
azithromycin
clarithromycin
dirithromycin
troleandomycin

These names are easy to recognize because they all end in "-omycin," and mostly in "-thromycin." Thus, they should be readily distinguishable from the amino-glycosides that end in "-mycin." Erythromycin and its relatives are generally well absorbed orally.

Erythromycin and it relatives are of particular use in the treatment of patients with *Mycoplasma* infections, pneumonia, Legionnaires disease, chlamydial infections, diphtheria, and pertussis.

Books vary somewhat as to their designation of erythromycin as the *drug of choice* for some of these diseases. Check your textbook or class notes and highlight those diseases that you need to know. Notice that many of these fall into the cat-egory of oddball infections.

Compare and contrast the tetracyclines and erythromycin. If you can't remember and someone asks the *drug of choice* for rickettsiae or Legionnaires dis-ease, guess tetracycline or erythromycin. Better yet, learn these few odd uses. One mnemonic that is sometimes used to remember the organisms for which eryth-romycin is the drug of choice is Legionnaires Camp on My Border (*Legionella, Campylobacter, Mycoplasma, Bordetella*).

The macrolides have few serious side effects—none that deserve a box of their own. GI upset is common, but you would have guessed that one, right?

There is a relatively new group of antibiotics, the ketolides, that were derived from the macrolides. The first is telithromycin. Notice that the name has the "mycin" ending. Bacteria that have developed resistance to macrolides are often still sensitive to ketolides. Telithromycin also has activity against intracellular respiratory pathogens.

STREPTOGRAMINS AND OXAZOLIDINONES

There are several new groups of protein synthesis inhibitors. One is the strepto-gramins. The first drug in this class is the combination of dalfopristin and quinupris-tin. The two components are always given together because they act synergistically to inhibit ribosome function.

The second group is the oxazolidinones—proudly represented by linezolid. These drugs inhibit protein synthesis by interfering with translation. The pre-dominant activity of linezolid is against aerobic gram-positive organisms and it is approved for vancomycin-resistant infections. It is also an inhibitor of monoamine oxidase. Reduction in MAO activity leads to an increase in the concentration of norepinephrine and can increase blood pressure.

The third group is actually a single drug (for now). Retapamulin is the first pleuromutilin available as an antibacterial agent. I'd suggest learning the name of the drug and not the name of the class. Retapamulin is derived from a fermentation produce of fungi. It interferes with the function of the 50S subunit of the bacterial ribosome.

Finally, mupirocin is a topical antibiotic originally isolated from a *Pseudomonas* that inhibits isoleucyl transfer RNA. Be sure to add any other new protein synthesis inhibitors to this section.

CHLORAMPHENICOL

Chloramphenicol is a broad-spectrum antibiotic, effective against most aerobic and anaerobic bacteria, except *Pseudomonas aeruginosa*.

> CHLORAMPHENICOL is associated with bone marrow depression and aplastic anemia that is usually *fatal*.

Chloramphenicol is reserved for life-threatening infections because of its serious, life-threatening adverse effects. A dose-related bone marrow depression can occur and a dose-related reversible anemia has been reported. An idiosyncratic aplastic anemia (1 in 40,000 cases) can occur that is usually *fatal*.

> CHLORAMPHENICOL can produce gray baby syndrome, which is often *fatal*.

Chloramphenicol is orally absorbed, penetrates the CSF, and is inactivated in the liver by conjugation. Infants have a decreased ability to conjugate chloramphenicol, resulting in high levels in the blood. They develop abdominal distention, vomiting, cyanosis, hypothermia, decreased respiration, and vasomotor collapse.

CLINDAMYCIN

These drugs (clindamycin and lincomycin) are sometimes called lincosamides based on their chemical structure. Notice that they end in "-mycin" but are not related to the aminoglycosides or macrolides. Lincomycin is rarely used, so focus on remembering clindamycin. The antibacterial activity of clindamycin is similar to that of erythromycin.

> Clindamycin penetrates most tissues, including bone. It has activity against anaerobes.

Clindamycin has been listed as the drug of choice for anaerobic GI infections. Use of clindamycin is associated with pseudomembranous colitis, because *Clostridium difficile* is resistant to clindamycin.

Folate Antagonists

CHAPTER 28

Mechanism of Action
Selected Features

MECHANISM OF ACTION

To understand the mechanism of action of this class of drugs, we need to first review the synthesis of folic acid (Figure 28–1). Bacteria cannot absorb folic acid, but must make it from PABA (para-aminobenzoic acid), pteridine, and glutamate. For humans, folic acid is a vitamin. We cannot synthesize it. This makes this metabolic pathway a nice, selective target for antimicrobial agents.

Sulfonamides and trimethoprim inhibit synthesis of folate at two different sites.

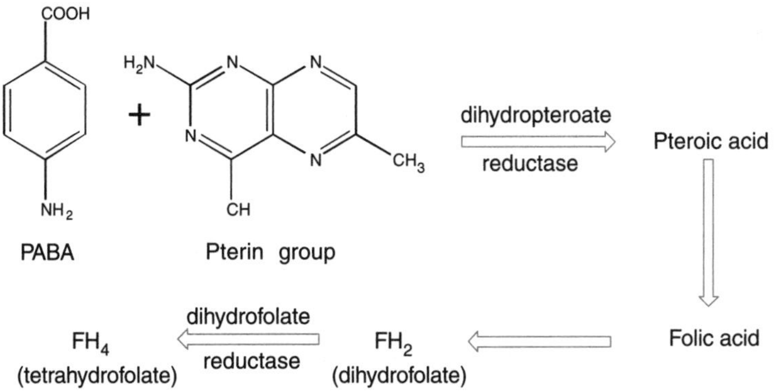

FIGURE 28–1 This figure presents the synthesis of folic acid, for review.

The sulfonamides are structurally similar to PABA and block the incorporation of PABA into dihydropteroic acid. Trimethoprim prevents reduction of dihydrofolate to tetrahydrofolate by inhibiting the enzyme dihydrofolate reductase. This enzyme is present in humans, but trimethoprim has a lower affinity for the human enzyme. There are other examples of folate reductase inhibitors that we will consider later (pyrimethamine and methotrexate).

The combination of sulfonamides and trimethoprim is synergistic, and they are rarely used alone. Sulfamethoxazole is the sulfonamide used in combination with trimethoprim because they have matching half-lives.

SULFAMETHOXAZOLE	sulfadiazine
TRIMETHOPRIM	sulfapyridine
cotrimoxazole	sulfasalazine
sulfacetamide	sulfisoxazole

There are other sulfonamides; please check your textbook. Note that sulfasalazine is also used to treat inflammatory bowel disease (see Chapter 42).

SELECTED FEATURES

These folate antagonists are broad-spectrum agents that are effective against gram-positive and gram-negative organisms.

The combination of sulfamethoxazole and trimethoprim, called cotrimoxazole, is probably the most commonly used drug in this group. It is used for urinary tract infections and *Pneumocystis carinii* pneumonitis, among other things.

Quinolones and Urinary Tract Antiseptics

> Drugs in This Group
> Quinolones
> Methenamine

DRUGS IN THIS GROUP

The quinolones are a group of relatively new antimicrobials that were originally used primarily to treat patients with urinary tract infections. Therefore, many books group these drugs together.

QUINOLONES

> **Quinolones**
> CIPROFLOXACIN
> enoxacin
> gemifloxacin
> gatifloxacin
> levofloxacin
> lomefloxacin
> ofloxacin
> moxifloxacin
> norfloxacin
> sparfloxacin
> trovafloxacin

For now, the names of the drugs in this class are easy to recognize. It is hoped the new ones that appear in the next few years will also be easy to recognize.

> The quinolones inhibit DNA synthesis through a specific action on DNA gyrase.

These drugs are considered in a separate category because they have a different structure and a different mechanism of action. They inhibit DNA gyrase and, thus, DNA synthesis. DNA gyrase is the bacterial enzyme that is responsible for unwinding and supercoiling of the DNA. This is the only class of antibacterials that inhibits DNA replication. This is a more common approach for the antivirals and the anticancer drugs.

> Quinolones are rarely first-line agents. They are used to treat genitourinary, respiratory, GI, and some skin and soft tissue infections.

These drugs are considered to be broad-spectrum antimicrobial agents. Nalidixic acid was the first available and it is an effective urinary tract antiseptic (it sterilizes the urine). The newer agents in this group are useful in a wide range of bacterial infections, including lower respiratory tract infections, bone and joint infections, and prostatitis. Some are effective against *Pseudomonas aeruginosa* and are orally active.

METHENAMINE

> Methenamine is metabolized to formaldehyde and ammonia and is used in urinary tract infections.

If you are simply overloaded at this point, skip this drug. Methenamine is an interesting example of a prodrug. The parent compound is not active. In acidic pH, it is hydrolyzed to ammonia and formaldehyde. The formaldehyde is lethal to bacteria. Therefore, this is another bactericidal drug. Methenamine is usually administered as a salt of an acid to help keep the pH of the urine less than 5.5, which is vital for the effective use of methenamine.

Drugs Used in Tuberculosis and Leprosy

Organization of Class
Isoniazid
Rifampin
Pyrazinamide
Ethambutol
Dapsone

ORGANIZATION OF CLASS

The mycobacteria that cause tuberculosis and leprosy are very slow growing, so therapy must be continued for relatively long periods of time. To prevent the emergence of resistant strains, it is vital to employ combination therapy with as many as four or five agents to which the organism is sensitive. The current treatment regimen for TB (which is subject to change) is 2 months of isoniazid, rifampin, pyrazinamide, and ethambutol, followed by 4 months of isoniazid and rifampin. Increasing the duration of therapy or changing the choice of drugs depends on culture and sensitivity results and factors that increase risk of treatment failure.

The drugs for TB are most commonly divided into two groups: first-line drugs and second-line drugs. For most purposes, knowledge of the first-line drugs is adequate. If you decide to specialize in infectious disease or the treatment of tuberculosis, then a working knowledge of the other drugs is important.

First-Line Drugs	Second-Line Drugs
ISONIAZID	amikacin
	aminosalicylic acid
PYRAZINAMIDE	capreomycin
RIFAMPIN	cycloserine
ethambutol	ethionamide
rifabutin	kanamycin
rifapentine	levofloxacin
	moxifloxacin
	streptomycin

Streptomycin was covered in more detail in Chapter 27, so we won't consider it again.

ISONIAZID

> ISONIAZID inhibits synthesis of mycolic acids.

Isoniazid has a very simple structure. It works on mycobacteria by inhibiting the synthesis of mycolic acids that are unique to the mycobacteria. The mycolic acids are constituents of the bacterial cell envelope.

> There are fast and slow acetylators of ISONIAZID.

You may have already heard mention of fast and slow acetylators. This is a genetically determined trait. Acetylation is a metabolic pathway for many drugs, but this pathway is of particular importance for isoniazid. Isoniazid has a shorter half-life in fast acetylators.

> ISONIAZID is associated with hepatotoxicity and peripheral neuropathy.

Hepatitis is the most severe side effect of isoniazid. Isoniazid-induced liver dysfunction (as measured by liver function tests) can occur in 10-20% of patients, and the incidence increases with age. The liver dysfunction is reversible in most patients.

The peripheral neuropathy results from pyridoxine deficiency. This deficiency results from a chemical combination of isoniazid and pyridoxine. It can be corrected by pyridoxine supplementation.

> ISONIAZID is the *drug of choice* for chemoprophylaxis in recent converters.

If a person has had negative TB tests (purified protein derivative [PPD] test) in the past, and then 1 year later the test is positive, that person is said to be a recent converter. The current recommendations (of course, subject to change) is that the person be placed on isoniazid for 9 months, as long as there is no evidence of clinical disease, such as a positive chest x-ray.

RIFAMPIN

> RIFAMPIN inhibits RNA synthesis by formation of a stable complex with the DNA-dependent RNA polymerase.

Rifampin binds to the β subunit of the enzyme, DNA-dependent RNA polymerase. The complex that is formed is inactive, thus blocking RNA synthesis. Resistance to rifampin is caused by a single-step mutation that results in an alteration of the β subunit. Not only is rifampin effective against tuberculosis, it is also effective against some gram-positive and gram-negative organisms.

> RIFAMPIN is metabolized in the liver and is a potent inducer of the P-450 enzymes. It can cause hepatitis and may color secretions red-orange.

Rifampin is deacetylated in the liver to an active metabolite. A drug-induced hepatitis can occur that results in jaundice. In addition, rifampin induces the liver microsomal P-450 enzymes. This can lead to increased metabolism of any other drug that is also metabolized by this system.

Rifampin may color urine, feces, saliva, sweat, and tears red-orange. The color can even get into contact lenses.

Rifabutin is an analogue of rifampin that has some activity against rifampin-resistant *Mycobacterium tuberculosis*.

PYRAZINAMIDE

> PYRAZINAMIDE is only effective against *M tuberculosis*. It increases levels of serum uric acid.

The mechanism of action of pyrazinamide is unknown. Pyrazinamide is particularly effective against intracellular organisms. Hyperuricemia occurs in all patients, but clinical gout is rare. Pyrazinamide has also been associated with hepatotoxicity.

ETHAMBUTOL

> Ethambutol can cause optic neuritis.

The mechanism of action of ethambutol is unknown, and it is the least potent of the first-line drugs. However, it has an interesting adverse effect that often appears on exams. Ethambutol can cause optic neuritis, resulting in loss of central vision and impaired red-green discrimination. Ethambutol may increase serum levels of uric acid as a result of decreased renal clearance of urate. The increased serum levels of uric acid may lead to gout.

DAPSONE

The treatment of leprosy is a very specialized area.

> DAPSONE is the mainstay in the treatment of leprosy.

For years dapsone was the mainstay of the treatment of patients with leprosy. However, worldwide, the problem of drug resistance is becoming severe. Therefore, current recommendations (again, subject to change) are that all forms of leprosy be treated with a combination of drugs. Dapsone is a structural analogue of PABA and is a competitive inhibitor of folic acid synthesis.

Rifampin is an active antileprosy drug as well as an anti-TB drug.

Interesting fact: The teratogenic drug, thalidomide, is the most effective drug for the treatment of erythema nodosum leprosum (an inflammatory reaction state associated with leprosy).

Antifungal Drugs

Organization of Class
Azole Antifungals
Polyene Antifungals
Echinocandins
Terbinafine

ORGANIZATION OF CLASS

Many fungal infections occur in poorly vascularized tissues or avascular structures such as the superficial layer of the skin, nails, and hair. Fungi are slow growing and are, therefore, more difficult to kill than bacteria, where cell division can be a target. Because many fungi are opportunistic, host factors play an important role in determining prognosis. The antifungal agents essentially assist the host immune system with the fight against the fungus.

In general these drugs are poorly soluble and, therefore, distribution to the site of action is often a problem. Consider these issues as you study these drugs. As with the antimicrobials, consider the issue of host versus invading organism. The drug should attack only the invading (foreign) organism and not the host (human) cells.

Classification can be done in a couple of ways. One of the most obvious ways to classify these drugs is by activity against systemic fungal infections or superficial fungal infections. The systemic infections include diseases such as disseminated blastomycosis or coccidioidomycosis. The superficial mycoses include infections with dermatophytes of the skin, hair, and nails.

A better way to organize the antifungals is by mechanism of action. Then, when new drugs are developed, you have a place to file the information in your brain.

Azoles		
imidazoles (2N)	topical and systemic	FLUCONAZOLE
topical	ketoconazole	ITRACONAZOLE
butoconazole	miconazole	VORICONAZOLE
clotrimazole	triazoles (3N)	posaconazole
econazole	systemic	terconazole
oxiconazole		

Polyenes	Others	Echinocandins
AMPHOTERICIN B	flucytosine	anidulafungin
nystatin	griseofulvin	caspofungin
	terbinafine	micofungin
	tolnaftate	

AZOLE ANTIFUNGALS

> The azoles are broad-spectrum fungistatic agents that inhibit the synthesis of ergosterol by inhibiting the 14-α-demethylase enzyme.

The azoles are so named because of the nitrogen containing azole ring structure that is part of each of these drugs (Figure 31–1). They are divided into two groups: the imidazoles with two nitrogens in the azole ring, and the triazoles with three nitrogens in the ring. Notice that the names all end in "-azole." This makes recognition of these agents easy.

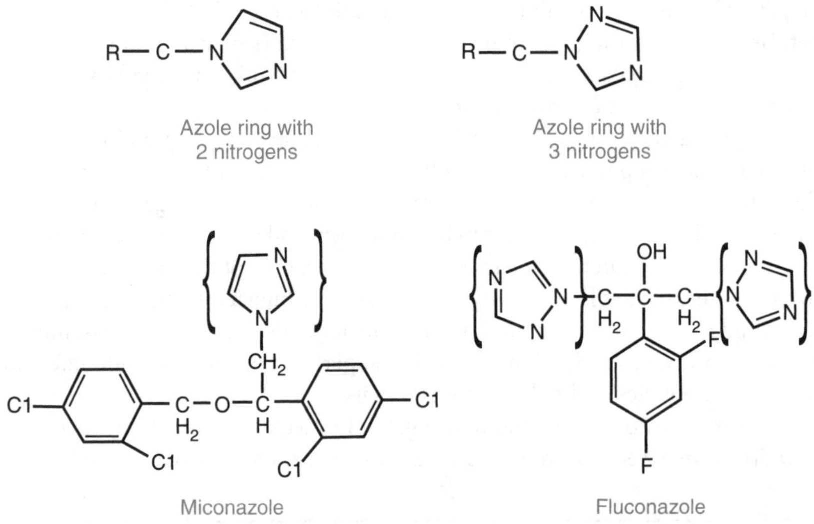

FIGURE 31–1 On the left are the imidazoles with two nitrogens in the azole ring, and on the right are the triazoles with three nitrogens in the azole ring.

Compared with the imidazoles, the triazoles tend to have fewer side effects, better drug distribution, and fewer drug interactions. Notice also that the imidazoles are primarily (although not exclusively) topical, whereas the triazoles are active systemically.

POLYENE ANTIFUNGALS

> The polyene antifungals, AMPHOTERICIN B and nystatin, work by binding to ergosterol, the principal fungal membrane sterol.

Amphotericin B is the antifungal agent that you should know better than the rest. However, remember that nystatin is also a polyene compound and has the same mechanism of action. Both drugs work by an interaction with ergosterol, the principal fungal membrane sterol. Mammalian cells also contain sterols (principally cholesterol). However, ergosterol has a greater affinity for amphotericin than does cholesterol. Once the drug has bound to the ergosterol, there is a disruption of membrane function and electrolytes can leak from the cell. Although it is not important to memorize the structures of any of these compounds, do take a moment to look at the structure of amphotericin B in Figure 31–2.

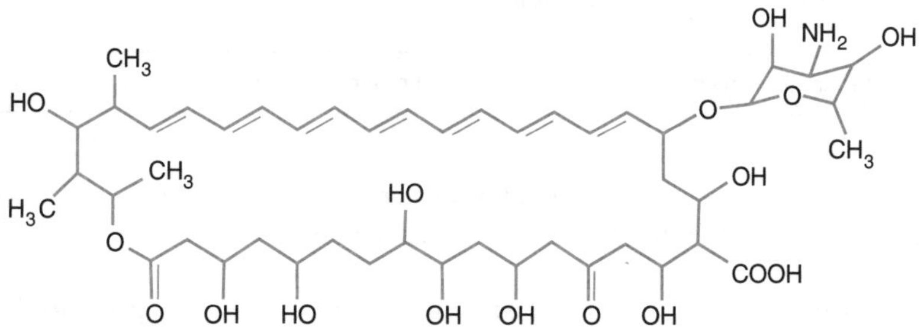

FIGURE 31–2 The structure of amphotericin B is shown here. Doesn't it look an awful lot like a lipid?

> AMPHOTERICIN B is most commonly used to treat serious disseminated yeast and fungal infections, particularly in immunocompromised patients.

Nystatin is too toxic for systemic use. Its use is limited to topical treatment for *Candida albicans*.

> The most serious and most common toxicity of AMPHOTERICIN B is nephrotoxicity.

Nephrotoxicity is related to dose and duration of therapy. Keeping patients well hydrated may reduce the nephrotoxicity. Fever, chills, and tachypnea occur commonly after the initial dose of amphotericin B. Amphotericin is now available in several lipid formulations in an attempt to reduce the toxicity.

> AMPHOTERICIN B is not absorbed from the gastrointestinal (GI) tract, so it must be given intravenously or topically.

ECHINOCANDINS

The echinocandins noncompetitively inhibit the synthesis of a major fungal cell wall component, β-(1,3)-D-glucan, which is not present in mammalian cell walls. Caspofungin, anidulafungin, and micofungin are all active against most *Candida* species and against the mold *Aspergillus*. All three drugs are given intravenously and appear to be similar in safety and efficacy. Note that, for now, the names all end in "-fungin."

TERBINAFINE

> Terbinafine is administered orally for treatment of superficial fungal infections.

The target tissues are those that are not well vascularized: hair, skin, and nails. Yet this drug is given orally and not applied topically.

> Terbinafine prevents ergosterol synthesis by inhibiting squalene epoxidase.

Terbinafine and tolnafatate inhibit squalene epoxidase, resulting in the accumulation of squalene inside the fungal cells. Terbinafine is effective against the skin and nail fungi.

Griseofulvin is an older, orally active drug used for dermatophyte infections.

Anthelmintic Drugs

Organization of Class

Drugs Used Against Cestodes and Trematodes

Drugs Used Against Nematodes

Drugs Used Against Filaria

ORGANIZATION OF CLASS

These drugs are effective against worms (helminths). In humans, the worms may remain within the intestinal lumen or may have complex life cycles that involve movement through the body. The infective form may be either an adult worm or an immature worm.

The worm life cycle is strongly dependent on neuromuscular coordination, energy production, and microtubular integrity. Most antiworm drugs target one of these three areas.

The easiest way to organize these drugs is to consider a reasonable organization of the worms. The helminths (worms) are classified into three groups: cestodes (flatworms), nematodes (roundworms), and trematodes (flukes). If you look at the table of worms and the drug of choice for each worm, several patterns emerge.

Helminth	Drug of Choice
Cestodes (flatworms and tapeworms)	PRAZIQUANTEL
Trematodes (flukes [schistosomiasis])	PRAZIQUANTEL
Nematodes	ALBENDAZOLE or MEBENDAZOLE
Roundworms (whip, pin, hook)	PYRANTEL
Filariasis	Diethylcarbamazine
	Ivermectin

DRUGS USED AGAINST CESTODES AND TREMATODES

PRAZIQUANTEL is the *drug of choice* for most trematode (fluke) and many cestode infections.

First, here's a quick review of the worms. Cestodes are the tapeworms. They are flat and segmented. The head has suckers. Larvae develop into adults in the small intestine. Therefore, treatment can be confined to the small intestine.

The trematodes are the flukes. If you recall, the flukes move about the body; there are blood flukes and liver flukes, and so on. Therefore, the treatment needs to reach the systemic circulation in order to affect the fluke.

The mechanism of action of praziquantel is unknown. It is postulated to alter membrane function of the worm and increase membrane permeability. It is absorbed after oral administration. That's why it can have an action on the trematodes (flukes) that cause schistosomiasis.

DRUGS USED AGAINST NEMATODES

> Treatment of nematodes (roundworms) consists of (for the most part) ALBENDAZOLE, MEBENDAZOLE, or PYRANTEL. The exception is filaria.

The nematodes are a more diverse set of worms. Overall, they are the roundworms because they are elongated and cylindrical (round). This group includes whipworm, pinworm, and hookworm. Most patients with nematode infections can be treated using mebendazole or pyrantel. A special group of nematodes can be considered separately: the filaria. Patients with filariasis are treated using two other drugs.

> ALBENDAZOLE and MEBENDAZOLE inhibit tubulin polymerization in the worms.

These drugs bind to β-tubulin and inhibit tubulin polymerization, which disrupts motility and replication. They can be given orally, and very little is absorbed from the gastrointestinal (GI) tract.

> PYRANTEL causes paralysis of the worms.

DRUGS USED AGAINST FILARIA

> Filariasis is treated (for the most part) with diethylcarbamazine or ivermectin.

Filaria are threadlike worms that are found in blood and tissue. They are transmitted by the bite of a fly or mosquito. Early in the infection, they move through the lymphatic system.

> Diethylcarbamazine is the *drug of choice* for lymphatic filariasis.

Diethylcarbamazine is not commercially available in the United States. This drug appears to alter the surface of the filaria in such a way that they are more susceptible to phagocytosis by the host immune system.

> Ivermectin paralyzes the worm muscle and is the *drug of choice* for onchocerciasis (cutaneous filariasis).

Ivermectin is more commonly known in veterinary medicine, but has found a niche in the treatment of onchocerciasis. It appears to block γ-aminobutyric acid (GABA)-mediated transmission in the invading organism without any effect on the host.

CHAPTER

33 Antiviral Drugs

Organization of Class
Anti-HIV Drugs
Drugs Used in Influenza
Other Antivirals

ORGANIZATION OF CLASS

Three basic approaches are taken to control viral diseases. Vaccination is used to try to prevent and control the spread of disease. Chemotherapy (the focus of pharmacology) is used to treat the symptoms of viral illness and to try to eliminate the virus from the body. Finally, stimulation of the host's natural resistance mechanisms is used to shorten the duration of illness.

The problems with chemotherapy are similar to those discussed for antimicrobial and antifungal agents. Anytime we are trying to kill an invading (foreign) organism, there is the problem of the drug recognizing and distinguishing the invading organism from the host. To understand the antiviral agents, it is necessary to review the life cycle of viruses and imagine sites where drugs could interfere or block:

1. Attachment and penetration of the virus to the host cell.
2. Uncoating of the viral genome within the host cell.
3. Synthesis of viral components within the host cell.
4. Assembly of viral particles.
5. Release of the virus to spread and invade other cells.

Most of the drugs that are currently available block specific viral proteins that are involved in synthesis of viral components within the host cell.

ANTI-HIV DRUGS

Reverse Transcriptase Inhibitors			Protease Inhibitors	Fusion and Entry Inhibitors
NRTIs	**NNRTIs**	**nucleotide**	atazanavir	enfuvirtide
abacavir	delavirdine	tenofovir	darunavir	maraviroc
didanosine	efavirenz		fosamprenavir	
emtricitabine	etravirine		indinavir	**Integrase Inhibitor**
lamivudine	nevirapine		lopinavir	raltegravir
stavudine			nelfinavir	
zidovudine			ritonavir	
			saquinavir	
			tipranavir	

As a reminder, human immunodeficiency virus (HIV), which is the virus that causes AIDS, is an RNA retrovirus. This means that it has a specific enzyme called reverse transcriptase. This is a major target of drugs with efficacy against HIV.

> The nucleoside (NRTIs), nucleotide, and nonnucleoside (NNRTIs) reverse transcriptase inhibitors (RT inhibitors) all inhibit the formation of viral DNA from RNA by reverse transcriptase.

The RT inhibitors are divided into several groups based on whether they are structurally related to nucleoside/nucleotides or not. The nucleoside analogues are related to thymidine and adenosine and, after triple phosphorylation, are incorporated into viral DNA during the reverse transcription of the viral RNA. But because they are not exactly the same as the native nucleosides, there is early termination of DNA elongation. The nucleotide RT inhibitor works in a similar manner, except that it is already phosphorylated once. The nonnucleoside inhibitors also stop the reverse transcriptase enzyme, but not by mimicking the natural nucleosides.

Mutation of the reverse transcriptase enzyme is very rapid. The use of at least two RT inhibitors simultaneously slows the emergence of resistant virus.

> The protease inhibitors interfere with processing of the viral protein, thus preventing formation of new viral particles.

The HIV protease enzyme is involved in maturation of the newly formed viral particle. These drugs have a number of side effects, including changes in fat deposition and metabolic abnormalities.

> Enfuvirtide blocks the fusion of the viral particle to the target cell, while maraviroc inhibits entry of the viral particles into cells.

Enfuvirtide is an analogue of the HIV protein that mediates fusion with the cell membrane. When enfuvirtide binds in place of the HIV protein it traps the viral particle in a conformation that prevents its fusion with the cell—thus the term fusion inhibitor. Enfuvirtide has to be given by injection. Maraviroc blocks one of the proteins (CCR5) that acts as a receptor for the HIV virus. Maraviroc is only active against HIV strains that are "R5 tropic."

> Raltegravir is the first available integrase inhibitor.

One key feature of HIV infection is that the virus integrates itself into the host cells genome, thus becoming part of the cell. This is mediated by a viral enzyme called integrase. Blocking this enzyme could potentially keep cells from becoming permanently infected with the HIV virus.

> Therapy for HIV is either based on inhibition of RT using one NNRTI + two NRTIs or based on use of a protease inhibitor using one or two PIs + two NRTIs.

DRUGS USED IN INFLUENZA

The mainstay of protection against influenza has always been vaccination. New drugs are now becoming available that effectively treat influenza.

Influenza Drugs	Neuraminidase Inhibitors
AMANTADINE	oseltamivir
rimantadine	peramivir (investigational)
	zanamivir

> AMANTADINE is used for the prevention and treatment of influenza type A infections.

If begun within 48 hours of the onset of illness, amantadine shortens the duration of symptoms by about half. The use of amantadine is limited by rapid emergence of resistance and by the drug's adverse effects.

> Neuraminidase inhibitors block release of influenza virus from infected cells.

A newer class, called neuraminidase inhibitors, works by inhibiting an enzyme located on the surface of the virus that breaks a bond between the virus and proteins on the cell surface, thus allowing formed viral particles to be released. The active site of the neuraminidase enzyme is a highly conserved site in both type A and type B influenza. The neuraminidase inhibitors bind to the active site and block it. Use of these agents is reported to shorten the duration of symptomatic illness if the drug is started within 30 hours of the onset of symptoms.

OTHER ANTIVIRALS

Other Antivirals

Herpes	RSV	Hepatitis B
ACYCLOVIR	RIBAVIRIN	adefovir
famciclovir	palivizumab	entecavir
ganciclovir		interferon-α
vidarabine (ara-A)		lamivudine
cidofovir		telbivudine
valacyclovir		
valganciclovir		

> ACYCLOVIR is used to treat patients with herpes infections. To be effective, it must be activated by triple phosphorylation.

Acyclovir is used topically, intravenously, and orally for the treatment of patients with herpes infections. As with the anti-HIV nucleoside RT inhibitors, acyclovir must undergo a triple phosphorylation to an active derivative. Acyclovir triphosphate inhibits the herpes virus DNA polymerase. A number of other "ciclovir" drugs are also used against herpes infections.

> RIBAVIRIN is used in the treatment of respiratory syncytial virus (RSV) in infants and young children.

The mechanism of action of ribavirin is unknown, but it is felt to be an antimetabolite. It is used in aerosol form for the treatment of RSV in young children. This could be labeled as a *drug of choice*. Palivizumab is a humanized monoclonal antibody against a glycoprotein on the surface of the virus. It is given as an injection at the start of RSV season in high-risk children to provide passive immunity.

Chronic hepatitis B is currently treated with weekly injections with interferon-α or daily oral treatment with a nucleoside analogue such as lamivudine or telbivudine. Hepatitis C is treated with interferon (peginterferon) and ribavirin.

CHAPTER

34

Antiprotozoal Drugs

Organization of Class
Metronidazole
Antimalarial Agents
Therapeutic Considerations
Special Features

ORGANIZATION OF CLASS

To simplify the discussion, the antimalarial drugs are covered in a separate section at the end of this chapter. Some of the more common protozoal diseases are listed in the following table.

Protozoa	Disease
Entamoeba histolytica	Amebiasis (diarrhea)
Balantidium coli	Balantidial dysentery
Trichomonas vaginalis	Trichomoniasis (genital infection)
Giardia lamblia	Giardiasis (diarrhea)
Leishmania	Leishmaniasis (three types)
Trypanosoma brucei	African sleeping sickness
Trypanosoma cruzi	Chagas disease (South American)

Of the drugs that are used in these diseases, metronidazole is the one that is the most important for you to know. Of the diseases listed, trichomoniasis and giardiasis are the most common in the United States and both are treated with metronidazole. This along with a few more details will go a long way. You need to be aware of the other drugs and where to find the information about treatment for these diseases.

Antiprotozoal Drugs

METRONIDAZOLE	nifurtimox
atovaquone	pentamidine
benznidazole	quinacrine
dehydroemetine	sodium stibogluconate
eflornithine	suramin
emetine	
iodoquinol	
melarsoprol	
meglumine antimonite	
nitazoxanide	

METRONIDAZOLE

> METRONIDAZOLE is effective in the treatment of vaginal trichomoniasis, giardiasis, and all forms of amebiasis.

Metronidazole is one of the most effective drugs against anaerobic bacteria and several protozoal species. It is highly effective in the treatment of trichomoniasis. It penetrates protozoal and bacterial cell walls, but cannot enter mammalian cells. The drug must be activated once it has entered the cell. The activating enzyme, nitroreductase, is only found in anaerobic organisms. The reduced metronidazole inhibits DNA replication by causing breaks and inhibiting repair of the DNA.

The most common side effects are nausea, vomiting, and diarrhea. The drug can turn the urine dark or red-brown and cause a metallic taste in the mouth. Metronidazole can cause a disulfiram-like reaction when taken with alcohol. The disulfiram-like effect consists of abdominal cramping, vomiting, flushing, or headache after drinking alcohol.

ANTIMALARIAL AGENTS

Malaria is caused by a single-cell protozoa, the plasmodium. There are over 50 species of plasmodia, but only four are infectious to humans: *Plasmodium malariae, Plasmodium ovale, Plasmodium vivax,* and *Plasmodium falciparum. Plasmodium vivax* is the most prevalent, but *P falciparum* is the most serious and lethal form of malaria.

To understand the drugs and the rationale behind treatment of patients with malaria, it is important to understand the life cycle of the malaria organism (Figure 34–1).

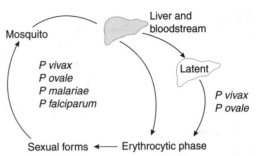

FIGURE 34-1 As a reminder, the life cycle of the malaria-causing protozoa is presented. *Plasmodium vivax* and *P ovale* are the two species that can take up residence in the liver.

Notice that only *P vivax* and *P ovale* can persist in the liver and, therefore, patients infected with these species can relapse.

THERAPEUTIC CONSIDERATIONS

It is thought that the symptoms are caused by the erythrocytic form of the parasite. Therefore, elimination of this asexual form will relieve symptoms. Drugs that do this are called suppressive or schizonticidal agents.

The emergence of chloroquine-resistant organisms is becoming a major health concern. However, the nuances of treatment of resistant organisms will not be addressed here. You should first try to understand the whys and wherefores of sensitive organisms. Later in your study of infectious disease, learn about the resistant organisms.

ANTI-MALARIAL DRUGS

CHLOROQUINE	hydroxychloroquine
PRIMAQUINE	mefloquine
QUININE	pyrimethamine
doxycycline	

To treat all strains, except those resistant to chloroquine, chloroquine is the oral drug of choice. That should be easy to remember. For parenteral use, quinidine and quinine are the drugs of choice. However, resistance is a major problem worldwide.

> Artemether-lumefantrine is highly effective for the treatment of uncomplicated malaria, including multidrug resistant infections.

Artemisinins are Chinese herbal products that have been shown to be quite effective against malaria. The active components are artemether and artesunate. Artemether inhibits nucleic acid and protein biosynthesis and is approved in the United States in combination with lumefantrine.

SPECIAL FEATURES

> PRIMAQUINE is effective against liver forms (exoerythrocytic) and kills gametocytes.

Because of its effectiveness against the liver phases, primaquine is often used for prophylaxis or prevention of relapse.

> PRIMAQUINE can cause hemolytic anemia in glucose-6-phosphate dehydrogenase (G6PD)–deficient patients.

Do you remember the G6PD enzyme? In biochemistry, you probably learned that some people are deficient in this enzyme and should avoid taking certain drugs. Primaquine is one of those drugs. This is an important (albeit somewhat specific) fact.

Chloroquine, in low doses, is not very toxic. However, in high doses or for long durations of treatment, it can cause toxicity of the skin, blood, and eyes. (Note: This is different from the standard nausea, vomiting, and diarrhea.) The drug becomes concentrated in melanin-containing structures and this can lead to corneal deposits and blindness.

The mechanism of action of quinine is unknown. It is derived from the bark of the cinchona tree, and the name given to describe quinine toxicity—cinchonism—reflects this. Cinchonism consists of sweating, ringing in the ears, impaired hearing, blurred vision, and N, V, D (nausea, vomiting, and diarrhea—for those of you who have not caught on).

Chloroquine is also used for prophylaxis for travelers entering areas where chloroquine-sensitive malaria is endemic.

35 Anticancer Drugs

Organization of Class
Terminology and General Principles of Therapy
Adverse Effects
Cytotoxic Drugs
    Alkylating Agents
    Antimetabolites
    Antibiotics and Other Natural Products
    Antibodies
    Other Cytotoxic Drugs
Hormonal Agents
Kinase Inhibitors
Miscellaneous Agents

ORGANIZATION OF CLASS

The anticancer drugs usually follow the antimicrobials in pharmacology text-books. This is because the drugs, in many cases, are similar.

Many students get really bogged down with the anticancer drugs. There are an awful lot of drugs with known mechanisms of action and multiple side effects that can be quite serious. However, there are some general principles of the use of these drugs that can be emphasized. In fact, these principles are more important than the individual agents. So, for the purposes of this book, focus on name recognition (be sure that you recognize a particular agent as an anticancer drug) and a few specific toxicities. Do not try to remember every type of cancer that the drug is used for. You can add some of this information later as you use these drugs in the clinical setting. Get a handle on the overall picture before you focus on the details.

> Many anticancer drugs have had several names over the years. Do not let this confuse you.

This is another very annoying thing about this group of drugs. Some of these agents are known by several names.

> *Cytotoxic drugs—drugs which block cell replication*
>   Alkylating agents, including nitrogen mustards and nitrosoureas
>   Antimetabolites, including folate antagonists, purine and pyrimidine analogues
>   Antibiotics and other natural products, including anthracyclines and vinca alkaloids
>   Antibodies—to improve specificity
>   Other cytotoxic drugs
> *Hormonal agents—drugs for hormone-sensitive tumors*
> *Miscellaneous agents*
>   Kinase inhibitors, including imatinib and gefitinib
>   Proteasome inhibitor—bortezomib

The drugs can be divided into two simple groups: the cytotoxic drugs and the hormones. All of the alkylating agents, antibiotics, antimetabolites, and miscellaneous drugs are cytotoxic drugs—they kill cells, particularly dividing cells. Therefore, all of the following terminology and general principles apply to the cytotoxic drugs. The hormonal agents are used for tumors of the hormonally sensitive tissues, such as breast and prostate. As always there are some drugs that do not fit neatly into these two categories.

TERMINOLOGY AND GENERAL PRINCIPLES OF THERAPY

> Anticancer therapy is aimed at killing dividing cells. There are normal host cells that are also dividing. Effects on these cells cause side effects.

This is a bit simplistic but serves our purposes for now. In antimicrobial therapy, the object is to kill the invading bacteria without harming the host. In anticancer therapy, the object is to kill the cancer cells without harming the normal cells. This is difficult because the cancer cells are also human (or host) cells. The cancer cells are basically human cells that have lost control of cell division. Therefore, anticancer treatment is, in large part, aimed at killing dividing cells. Remember that cells in certain places in the body—the epithelium of the gastrointestinal (GI) tract, hair follicles, and bone marrow, especially—are dividing continuously. Effects on these dividing cells cause adverse effects.

Because many of these drugs target dividing cells, the cell cycle is important to remember (Figure 35–1). When known, textbooks will list the part of the cell cycle in which a drug has an effect or they will list that a drug is cell cycle-specific or not. This is not absolutely critical information for your first pass through the material. However, as you learn more about the tumors and their growth rates, this information should be added.

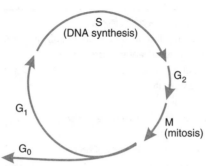

FIGURE 35–1 Cells go through several cycles around cell division. DNA synthesis occurs during the S phase and the actual division takes place during the M phase.

> The log kill is an important concept to understand. The anticancer drugs kill a constant fraction of cells instead of an absolute number.

The anticancer drugs act by first-order kinetics (Figure 35–2). Remember kinetics? This means that a constant fraction of the cells (say, 50%) are killed by one dose. This is quite different from a constant number of cells being killed. If one dose of the drug kills 50% of the tumor cells, then a second dose of the drug will kill 50% of the remaining tumor cells. This results in a 75% reduction in the number of tumor cells after two doses of this drug. This sort of thinking should remind you very much of pharmacokinetics. The number of tumor cells is usually expressed in exponentials. This is why the so-called kill of a drug is described in log units. The drug that reduces the tumor cell load from 10^8 cells to 10^5 cells is said to have achieved a "3 log kill."

> Drug resistance to anticancer drugs is analogous to resistance to antimicrobials.

Cancer cells already contain a mutation that allows unrestricted growth. They can also mutate in a way that makes them resistant to anticancer drugs.

> Combinations of drugs are frequently used in the treatment of cancer.

Combinations of drugs are frequently used to treat cancer. This reduces the incidence of drug resistance. In addition, the drugs used together often target different phases of the cell cycle or one of the drugs is non–cell cycle specific. The common drug combinations often have acronyms, such as MOPP, VAMP, or POMP, which stand for the individual drugs in the combination. It is not necessary at this time to learn the drug combinations.

ADVERSE EFFECTS

As previously mentioned, the adverse effects of these drugs result from their effects on proliferating cells in the body. We will consider the toxicity of these drugs separately, because the principles behind the toxicity are more important than remembering which drugs have more, or less, of a particular toxicity.

> Bone marrow toxicity is caused by destruction of proliferating hematopoietic stem cells. This results in a decrease in all blood elements, including white cells and platelets.

Patients receiving anticancer drugs are at increased risk of developing life-threatening infections and bleeding. This is due to the decrease in white blood cells and platelets. Growth factors are now available that can be used to stimulate cell production in the bone marrow. Fil*gra*stim (granulocyte colony-*stim*ulating factor) is used to accelerate recovery of neutrophils and sar*gramo*stim (granulo-cyte-*macro*phage colony-*stim*ulating factor) is used to accelerate bone marrow repopulation after chemotherapy, radiation, and bone marrow transplantation. Thrombopoietin and erythropoietin can be used to stimulate formation of plate-lets and red blood cells, respectively. Plerixafor, a CXCR4 chemokine receptor antagonist, can be used in combination with granulocyte colony-stimulating fac-tor to mobilize peripheral stem cells.

> Gastrointestinal toxicity takes two forms. The nausea and vomiting associated with can-cer chemotherapy is felt due to a central effect. These drugs can also directly damage the proliferating mucosa of the GI tract.

Almost all of the cancer chemotherapy drugs cause nausea and vomiting (of course, some are worse than others). It is felt that the drugs stimulate the chemoreceptor trigger zone in the brain that leads to vomiting. Serotonin antago-nists (specifically 5-HT$_3$), such as ONDANSETRON, dolasetron, granisetron, and palonosetron, have also proved effective in the prevention of nausea and vomit-ing. (Notice that they all end in "-setron.") A different type of antiemetic is the substance P neurokinin-1 receptor antagonist, aprepitant. Neurokinin-1 receptors are present in the emesis center in the medulla. Protection against vomiting can be enhanced by using both 5-HT$_3$ and neurokinin-1 antagonists in combination with a glucocorticoid. A synthetic cannabinoid (nabilone) is also available for the treatment of chemotherapy-induced nausea and vomiting.

The more predictable effect of the anticancer drugs is killing the proliferating cells in the mucosa of the GI tract. Remember that the epithelium of the GI tract is constantly replicating. These drugs kill dividing cells. Therefore, they will damage the epithelium of the GI tract. This can lead to ulcer formation anywhere in the GI tract—mouth, esophagus, stomach, and so on.

> Most anticancer drugs damage hair follicles and produce hair loss.

This is especially true with cyclophosphamide, doxorubicin, vincristine, methotrexate, and dactinomycin. (Do not worry too much about this for now.)

> Renal tubular damage is the major side effect of cisplatin and high-dose methotrexate. Cyclophosphamide can cause hemorrhagic cystitis.

Renal damage is not that common after use of the anticancer drugs. However, it is a significant side effect of a few drugs. So, learn these few. For many of the drugs, adequate hydration is recommended. But details like these should be added later.

> Cardiotoxicity is associated with the use of doxorubicin and daunorubicin (the anthracyclines).

Cardiotoxicity is relatively rare with the anticancer drugs. However, there are two drugs that stand out in this category—the two "D-rubicins." This particular adverse effect has a habit of showing up on board examinations and other such places.

> Bleomycin can cause pulmonary fibrosis, which can be *fatal*.

This is another example of a particular drug–adverse effect pair that has a habit of showing up in the most unusual locations. It's not too hard to memorize.

> Vincristine is known for its nervous system toxicity.

Vincristine is the only anticancer drug that has a dose-limiting neurotoxicity. Anytime we can use the word *only*, it should register on a memory chip in your brain.

CYTOTOXIC DRUGS

ALKYLATING AGENTS

> Alkylating agents all work by adding an alkyl group to DNA.

These drugs all introduce alkyl groups into nucleophilic sites with covalent bonds. There are many sites of alkylation, but the degree of DNA alkylation correlates with the cytotoxicity of the drugs. These drugs are not cycle specific. They are prone to cause local tissue necrosis and damage.

A. *Nitrogen mustards*	C. *Other alkylating agents*
Bendamustine	Busulphan
Chlorambucil	Carboplatin
Cyclophosphamide	Cisplatin
Ifosfamide	Oxaliplatin
Mechlorethamine (nitrogen mustard)	Dacarbazine
Melphalan	Temozolomide
B. *Nitrosoureas*	Thiotepa
Carmustine	
Lomustine	

The nitrosoureas are easy to recognize because of the "-mustine" ending on their names. They are lipid soluble and therefore cross into the central nervous system (CNS). They have found use in the treatment of brain tumors.

The other alkylating agents—well, if you can remember the names—great.

ANTIMETABOLITES

The antimetabolites compete for binding sites on enzymes or can be incorporated into DNA or RNA. They are especially useful if they bind to an enzyme that has a major effect on pathways leading to cell replication. That should make sense.

> Methotrexate competitively inhibits dihydrofolate reductase.

Remember this pathway from the discussion of folate antagonists? (See Figure 28–1.) Well, methotrexate inhibits the binding of folic acid to the enzyme. It therefore inhibits DNA synthesis by inhibiting thymidylate synthesis. Cellular uptake of methotrexate is by a carrier-mediated active transport. Cellular resistance to methotrexate is presumably caused by decreased transport into the cell. This can be overcome by using high doses.

> Leucovorin provides reduced folate to "rescue" normal cells from the action of methotrexate.

Even before you took pharmacology, you had probably heard of leucovorin rescue during cancer treatment. Leucovorin provides cells with reduced folate, thus bypassing the blocked enzyme.

> Methotrexate is used to treat psoriasis and severe rheumatoid arthritis in addition to a whole variety of cancers. It can be administered intrathecally.

The other drugs in this group mimic purines or pyrimidines. They get incorporated into the growing DNA during cell division and block further DNA replication. Thus, they are most effective in dividing cells.

A. *Purine analogues*
    cladribine
    fludarabine
    mercaptopurine (6-mercaptopurine)
    pentostatin
    thioguanine (6-thioguanine)

B. *Pyrimidine analogues*
    capecitabine (prodrug for 5-FU)
    cytarabine (cytosine arabinoside, ara-C)
    fluorouracil (5-FU)
    gemcitabine

The purine and pyrimidine analogues all have to be activated (phosphorylated) before they are effective.

Compare this activation to that of the antivirals (see Chapter 33).

A. *Anthracyclines*
    daunorubicin (daunomycin)
    doxorubicin
    epirubicin
    idarubicin
B. *Other antibiotics*
    bleomycin
    dactinomycin (actinomycin D)
    mitomycin (mitomycin C)
    plicamycin (mithramycin)

C. *Vinca alkaloids*
    vinblastine
    vincristine
    vinorelbine
D. *Other natural products*
    docetaxel
    paclitaxel
    Etoposide
    Teniposide
    Irinotecan

ANTIBIOTICS AND OTHER NATURAL PRODUCTS

As you can see, there are an awful lot of drugs. Notice that under the antibiotics and natural products, there are a number of drugs that end in "-mycin." Be careful not to confuse these with the antibiotics that have the same ending.

The antibiotics all disrupt DNA function.

Most of these drugs bind in some way to DNA. It is easiest to divide the antibiotics into two groups: the anthracyclines and the others.

The anthracyclines have cardiac toxicity.

The anthracyclines are so named because of their structure. However, the structure is not of primary importance to us. The cardiac toxicity is the most important thing to know about the "-rubicins." Highlight it, make a flash card, do whatever it takes to get you to remember this. The cardiac problems include arrhythmias, decreased function, myofibrillar degeneration, and focal necrosis of myocytes. It is felt that clinical cardiac damage occurs with each dose. It has been postulated that the damage is caused by free radical generation and lipid peroxidation. There is a drug available to help protect the cardiac muscle from this anthracycline-induced toxicity—dexrazoxane. Dexrazoxane chelates intracellular iron. Then the iron cannot react with superoxide anions and hydrogen peroxide to produce the highly toxic-free radicals.

Now on to the other antibiotics, the "-mycins."

> Bleomycin can cause *fatal* pulmonary fibrosis. It does not have significant myelosuppressive effects.

> Plicamycin (mithramycin) can be used to treat life-threatening hypercalcemia associated with malignancy.

Plicamycin inhibits resorption of bone by osteoblasts, thus lowering serum calcium. This fact also appears in the oddest of places.

Let's move on to the other plant products, or naturally occurring agents.

> The vinca alkaloids (vincristine, vinblastine, and vinorelbine) bind to tubulin and disrupt the spindle apparatus during cell division.

These three drugs are the most important ones for you to know.

> For vincristine, the neurological toxicity is dose-limiting. For vinblastine and vinorelbine, the bone marrow toxicity is dose-limiting.

If you can remember that one has neurological toxicity and the other two have bone marrow toxicity, then notice that vinblastine and vinorelbine (the ones with the "b" in the name) are bone marrow toxic.

> Paclitaxel works by preventing depolymerization of microtubules.

Paclitaxel is isolated from the rare Pacific yew tree and quantities are very limited. Docetaxel is synthesized from a precursor isolated from the more available European yew tree. Ixabepilone is a semisynthetic drug that also binds to microtubules, so while it's not included in the list of natural products, it deserves a mention here.

> Etoposide, teniposide, and irinotecan are plant products that inhibit topoisomerase.

These three drugs are further down on the trivia list. Learn the names if you have time and energy. They are noted here so that you do not generalize the tubulin action to all the natural plant products.

ANTIBODIES

In order to improve specificity in the treatment of cancer, a number of antibodies have been developed that target proteins expressed on the tumor cells. Samples of these antibodies are presented in the following table—along with the protein target for the antibody.

alemtuzumab—CD52
bevacizumab—VEGFR
cetuximab—EGFR
gemtuzumab ozogamicin—CD33
ibritumomab tiuxetan labeled with yttrium 90—CD20
lapatinib—HER2 and EGFR-1
ofatumumab—CD20
panitumumab—EGFR
rituximab—CD20
tositumomab labeled with I-131—CD20
trastuzumab—HER2

Notice that two of the listed antibodies for CD20 (a B cell antigen) have a radioactive label. The antibody brings the radiation to the tumor cells to increase specificity of the radiation. Ibritumomab tiuxetan is a combination molecule. The antibody is the ibritumomab piece that is bonded to the chelator tiuxetan. The chelator provides the binding site for the radioactive ligand.

Gemtuzuman ozogamicin is a monoclonal antibody to the CD33 antigen, which is expressed on the surface of leukemic myeloblasts and immature cells of the myelomonocytic line, conjugated with an antitumor antibiotic called calicheamicin. The binding of the antibody to the surface of the cell triggers internalization of the complex. The calicheamicin piece is released and binds to DNA causing the strand to break. Thus, this antibody improves targeting of a cytotoxic agent.

OTHER CYTOTOXIC DRUGS

asparaginase
hydroxyurea
mitotane
mitoxantrone
procarbazine (*N*-methyl-hydrazine, alkylating)

There are numerous other anticancer drugs. Some of these are occasionally classified as alkylating agents (procarbazine). Please compare the earlier listing to that in your textbook or class handouts.

Hydroxyurea inhibits ribonucleotide reductase.

Mitotane is used to treat adrenocortical adenocarcinoma.

HORMONAL AGENTS

A. *Glucocorticoids*
B. *Aromatase inhibitors*
   anastrozole
   exemestane
   formestane
   letrozole
C. *Estrogens/antiestrogens*
   fulvestrant
   tamoxifen citrate
   toremifine

D. *Androgen receptor antagonists*
   bicalcutamide
   flutamide
   nilutamide
E. *GnRH analogues and antagonists*
   abarelix (antagonist)
   degarelix (antagonist)
   gosrelin (analogue)
   leuprolide (antagonist/analogue)
   triptorelin (analogue)

These drugs are used to treat hormonally sensitive tumors, such as tumors of the breast, prostate, and uterus. The side effects of the drugs are related to the hormonal changes that they induce and not to cytotoxic actions. The goal is to (1) reduce the levels of the hormone that is stimulating growth of the tumor or (2) block the receptor for the hormone.

> Aromatase inhibitors block estrogen formation and are used to treat estrogen-dependent tumors (breast cancer) resistant to tamoxifen.

Estrogen is synthesized from androgen precursors by an enzyme called aromatase. Therefore, inhibiting this enzyme will reduce the production of estrogen. Anastrozol and letrozole are competitive inhibitors of aromatase. Notice that they are *not* "azoles," which are antifungal drugs, but they are both "*ozoles*." Exemestane and formestane (the "mestanes") bind covalently to the enzyme.

> Tamoxifen and toremifene are competitive antagonists of the estrogen receptor, used in the treatment of breast cancer.

In addition to the competitive antagonists of the estrogen receptor, fulvestrant also works as an estrogen-receptor antagonist. However, in contrast to tamoxifen it downregulates the estrogen receptor.

> The "lutamides" are competitive testosterone antagonists that are used to treat prostate cancer.

> Both GnRH analogues and antagonists will decrease serum levels of estrogen and testosterone and are used to treat androgen-dependent prostate cancer.

The hypothalamus normally releases gonadotropin-releasing hormone (GnRH) in a pulsatile fashion. Continuous administration of a GnRH analogue (one of the "relins") will suppress release of leutinizing hormone (LH) and follicle-stimulating hormone (FSH) and, as a result, decrease estrogen and testosterone levels, but there may be an initial surge in hormone levels before the decline. Antagonists of GnRH receptors will have the same effect, but will cause an inmmediate decrease in hormone levels. The GnRH analogues and antagonists are used in the treatment of androgen-dependent prostate cancer.

KINASE INHIBITORS

There is a relatively new group of anticancer drugs called signal transduction inhibitors. Instead of a focus on DNA replication or cell division, these drugs target cell signaling transduction mechanisms. For example, there are now a whole group of tyrosine kinase inhibitors. Since they are mediators of cell growth, differentiation and death, the activity of tyrosine kinases are normally very tightly regulated.

Imatinib was the first kinase inhibitor to be developed. In some patients with chronic myelogenous leukemia, the chromosomal translocation (Philadelphia chromosome) results in the formation of a tyrosine kinase that the cell cannot regulate (constitutively active). Imatinib binds to the ATP site on the newly formed kinase and can stop the growth of cells that contain this abnormal kinase. Normal cells are not affected. It is also useful against gastrointestinal stromal tumors. The discovery of the imatinib opened the door to the testing and development of other kinase inhibitors for a variety of cancers. Notice the "nib" ending of these names.

> dasatinib—multikinase inhibitor
> everolimus—mTOR inhibitor
> gefitinib—EGFR tyrosine kinase inhibitor
> erlotinib—EGFR tyrosine kinase inhibitor
> imatinib—BCR-abl kinase inhibitor
> nilotinib—BCR-abl kinase inhibitor
> pazopanib—multikinase inhibitor
> sunitinib—multikinase inhibitor
> sorafenib—multikinase inhibitor
> temsirolimus—mTOR inhibitor

Agents that prevent tumor proliferation through inhibition of the vascular endothelial growth factor receptor (EGFR) or the mammalian target of rapamycin (mTOR) pathway have become standard care in some cancers. The mTOR inhibitors are also used to prevention rejection after transplant. The multikinase inhibitors block kinases that are important in cellular signaling cascades involved in tumor proliferation or angiogenesis (growth of new blood vessels).

MISCELLANEOUS AGENTS

Bortezomib is a proteosome inhibitor. The proteasome is a large complex of proteins that is responsible for the regulation of protein expression and the degradation of damaged or used proteins in the cell. Importantly, it regulates the expression of cell cycle proteins. Happily, malignant cells are more sensitive to inhibition of proteosome function than normal cells.

Agents such as retinoids stimulate the growth of normal myeloid and erythroid progenitors and cause differentiation of myeloid leukemic cells. Clinical trials have shown that transretinoic acid (tretinoin) induces remission in acute promyelocytic leukemia.

A couple a histone deacetylase (HDAC) inhibitors (romidepsin and vorinostat) have been approved for the treatment of cutaneous T-cell lymphoma. HDAC inhibitors cause acetylated nuclear histones to accumulate in both tumor and normal tissues. In addition, acetylated transcription factors are also found. The precise mechanism of the anticancer activity of HDAC inhibitors is an area of active research. In early studies, HDAC inhibitors have shown significant efficacy and safety and they are being investigated for other disease besides cancer.

PART VI Drugs That Affect the Endocrine System

CHAPTER 36: Adrenocortical Hormones   185

CHAPTER 37: Sex Steroids   189

CHAPTER 38: Thyroid and Parathyroid Drugs   196

CHAPTER 39: Insulin, Glucagon, and Oral Hypoglycemic Drugs   199

Adrenocortical Hormones

Organization of Class
Glucocorticoids
Mineralocorticoids
Inhibitors of Adrenocorticoid Synthesis

ORGANIZATION OF CLASS

The term *steroid* relates to the main structural frame of this series of compounds (Figure 36–1).

The steroid compounds produced by the adrenal cortex are called adrenocorticosteroids, and they can be divided into two main groups depending on their relative metabolic (glucocorticoid) versus electrolyte-regulating (mineralocorticoid) activity. Of course, each compound has effects on both metabolism and electrolyte balance, but one effect is usually more potent than the other. Almost every cell in the body will respond to these compounds.

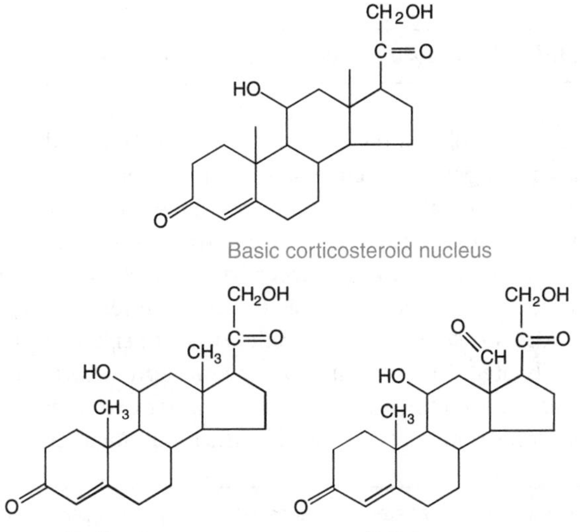

FIGURE 36–1 The main steroid structure is shown, along with two examples of adrenocortical hormones.

glucocorticoid	Equal Potency	Mineralocorticoid
DEXAMETHASONE	cortisol	fludrocortisone
PREDNISONE	hydrocortisone	
fluticasone		
betamethasone		
methylprednisolone		
prednisolone		
triamcinolone		

Compare this list of drugs with the list in your textbook or class handouts and make any necessary changes. I have found lists of more than 20 glucocorticoids, so the table above is quite abbreviated.

> HYDROCORTISONE (CORTISOL) is the main glucocorticoid produced by the adrenal glands.

Notice that hydrocortisone and its close relative, cortisol, are the *only* two drugs that have equal metabolic (glucocorticoid) and electrolyte balance (mineralocorticoid) actions. Remember this. Next, notice that there are many more drugs listed on the left (glucocorticoid) than on the right (mineralocorticoid). Therefore, if you have to guess about the activity of a drug, guess glucocorticoid. Better yet, just learn the mineralocorticoid drug on the right (it starts with "f," but it's not the only one that does).

> Aldosterone is the main mineralocorticoid produced by the adrenal glands.

It is useful at this point to review some of the anatomy and physiology of the adrenal gland, with a particular emphasis on the adrenal cortex (Figure 36–2). Remember that the adrenal medulla produces epinephrine and norepinephrine. Within the adrenal cortex, there are three layers. The zona glomerulosa (outer layer) produces the compounds that control electrolyte balance, such as aldosterone. The zona fasciculata (middle layer) produces the compounds that regulate metabolism, such as hydrocortisone. The zona reticularis (inner layer) produces the sex hormones (see Chapter 37). The pituitary hormone adrenocorticotropic hormone (ACTH) controls the secretion of, primarily, the inner two layers. The production of mineralocorticoids is mainly controlled by the renin-angiotensin system.

> The pharmacological actions of steroids are an extension of their physiological effects.

This should seem self-evident, but sometimes it is forgotten.

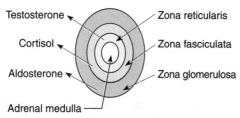

Testosterone — Zona reticularis

Cortisol — Zona fasciculata

Aldosterone — Zona glomerulosa

Adrenal medulla —

FIGURE 36–2 This figure reminds you of the layers of the adrenal cortex and the hormones that each layer produces.

> All of the steroids (including the sex steroids) bind to intracellular receptors in target tissues.

After entering the cell and binding to the receptor, the receptor-hormone complex is transported into the nucleus where it acts as a transcription factor for specific genes. The actions of the glucocorticoids and mineralocorticoids will be reviewed separately.

GLUCOCORTICOIDS

Glucocorticoid receptors are found in virtually every cell in the body.

> Glucocorticoids promote catabolism of proteins and gluconeogenesis.

The glucocorticoids stimulate formation of glucose and cause breakdown of proteins into amino acids. The net effect is to increase liver glycogen levels, fasting blood glucose levels, and urinary nitrogen output.

> Glucocorticoids inhibit inflammatory and immunological responses. This is the basis of their therapeutic use and the reason why patients on glucocorticoids have increased susceptibility to infections.

Glucocorticoids are used for replacement therapy in patients with malfunctioning adrenal glands. But the most important use of glucocorticoids is to reduce inflammation or block immunological and allergic responses. All steps in the inflammatory process are blocked.

Glucocorticoids have a number of other actions. You should read about them, but do not try to memorize them early on. Remember that these compounds affect nearly every cell in the body.

> The complications of glucocorticoid therapy appear in all organ systems.

This should be intuitive. Because the glucocorticoids affect nearly every cell in the body, the adverse effects can arise from nearly every cell in the body.

Short-term use (for example, in status asthmaticus) is generally safe. It is long-term use that poses particular problems.

> A potentially serious complication of long-term use is osteoporosis.

Glucocorticoids affect bone metabolism in a number of ways. The final result is a decrease in calcification. With long-term therapy, redistribution of fat also occurs, resulting in truncal obesity, moon facies, and buffalo hump. The effects on protein metabolism cause delayed wound healing.

MINERALOCORTICOIDS

> Mineralocorticoids are involved in salt and water balance.

Mineralocorticoids increase the rate of sodium, bicarbonate, and water reabsorption and potassium excretion. These actions help maintain normal concentrations of sodium and potassium in the serum.

INHIBITORS OF ADRENOCORTICOID SYNTHESIS

This group of drugs is used clinically to treat the glucocorticoid overproduction that appears in some diseases (Cushing disease, adrenal carcinoma, and others).

Metyrapone and aminoglutethimide inhibit adrenalcorticoid synthesis. Name recognition is the most important thing here. If you have the time and energy, add the mechanisms of action.

Aminoglutethimide and metyrapone inhibit the conversion of cholesterol to pregnenolone by an enzyme called 11-β-hydroxylase (the rate-limiting step in steroid synthesis). Ketoconazole, an antifungal agent, and spironolactone, an antagonist of aldosterone, also inhibit adrenal hormone synthesis.

Sex Steroids

Organization of Class

Estrogens

Antiestrogens

Progestins

Antiprogestins

Oral Contraceptives

Androgens

Antiandrogens

GnRH agonists and antagonists

PDE5 Inhibitors

ORGANIZATION OF CLASS

Sex hormones are produced by the gonads and inner layer of the cortex of the adrenal medulla. The synthesis and release of the hormones are controlled by the anterior pituitary (luteinizing hormone [LH] and follicle-stimulating hormone [FSH]) and the hypothalamus (gonadotropin-releasing hormone). Therefore, we are including in this chapter the actual sex steroids, but also GnRH agonists and antagonists.

Estrogens	Antiestrogens
DIETHYLSTILBESTROL	CLOMIPHENE
ESTRADIOL	TAMOXIFEN
estriol	RALOXIFENE
estrone	toremifene
ethinyl estradiol	
mestranol	
quinestrol	

(Continued)

Progestins	Antiprogestins
PROGESTERONE	MIFEPRISTONE
hydroxyprogesterone	
medroxyprogesterone	
megestrol	
norethindrone	
norgestrel	
levonorgestrol	

Androgens	Antiandrogens
TESTOSTERONE	Dutasteride (5α-*reductase inhibitors*)
(several preparations)	FINASTERIDE
Fluoxymesterone	Flutamide *(receptor antagonist)*
Methyltestosterone	Cyproterone acetate
Testolactone	**N**ilutamide

First, compare these drug names to those in your textbook or class handouts. The androgens listed here are only the androgenic steroids. I have not included the agents used primarily as anabolic agents. Look at each name and decide whether you recognize it for what it is. (That is, do you know that norgestrel is a progestin?) Put those you are not sure of in your list for name recognition. The rest of this is easy, especially if you remember your endocrine physiology (Figure 37–1).

As with the glucocorticoids, the sex steroids bind to specific intracellular receptors that are nuclear transcription factors.

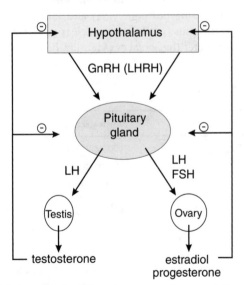

FIGURE 37–1 This is a very simplified scheme to remind you of the regulation of the sex steroids. There are additional positive and negative feedback mechanisms to the pituitary. GnRH is gonadotropin-releasing hormone, which is sometimes called LH-RH (luteinizing hormone–releasing hormone).

ESTROGENS

> The major estrogens produced by the body are estradiol, estrone, and estriol.

The ovary is the primary source of estradiol. Estrone and estriol are metabolites of estradiol, courtesy of the liver.

> The most common use of estrogens is in oral contraceptives.

Estrogen therapy combined with progestins is used to block ovulation and prevent pregnancy. In postmenopausal women, estrogens can be used to reduce the symptoms of menopause and osteoporosis. Hormone replacement therapies can slow bone loss, but cannot reverse existing deficits. However, there is now evidence that the risks of estrogen-replacement therapy may outweigh the benefits.

> The most common side effects of estrogens are nausea and vomiting.

Estrogens can also cause breast tenderness, endometrial hyperplasia, hyperpigmentation, edema (sodium and water retention), and weight gain.

> DIETHYLSTILBESTROL (a nonsteroid molecule) has been associated with cervical and vaginal carcinoma in daughters of women who take the drug during pregnancy.

ANTIESTROGENS

There are two important groups of drugs that antagonize the action of estrogen—the SERMS and clomiphene.

> The selective estrogen receptor modulators (SERM) are not pure antagonists, but mixed agonists/antagonists.

Tamoxifen and toremifene are used in the prevention and treatment of breast cancer that has estrogen receptors and is covered in more detail in Chapter 35. These drugs are antagonists in breast tissue and partial agonists in bone and endometrial tissue. Raloxifene has agonist activity in bone, but antagonist activity in breast and endometrial tissue. Raloxifene is approved for treatment of postmenopausal osteoporosis (see Chapter 45).

> CLOMIPHENE stimulates ovarian function and is used in the treatment of infertility.

Clomiphene acts as an estrogen receptor antagonist in the hypothalamus, thus interfering with the inhibitory feedback of estrogens. This results in an increase in release of gonadotropin-releasing hormone and gonadotropins and in stimulation of ovarian function.

PROGESTINS

> PROGESTERONE is the main natural progestin.

Progesterone is produced in the corpus luteum and placenta. Its job is to maintain the uterine endometrium in the secretory phase.

> The major use of progestins is in oral contraceptives.

Other clinical uses of progestins include dysfunctional uterine bleeding, suppression of postpartum lactation, treatment of dysmenorrhea, and management of endometriosis.

> The most common side effects of progestin use are weight gain, edema, and depression.

Increased clotting may also occur, leading to thrombophlebitis or pulmonary embolism.

ANTIPROGESTINS

> MIFEPRISTONE is an antiprogestin that works to terminate pregnancy by breaking down the uterine lining.

The current regimen for medical abortion is a multistep process. Mifepristone is administered first, followed 2 days later by misoprostol (see Chapter 42). As an antiprogestin, mifepristone can also be used to treat cases of infertility, endometriosis, and some tumors. It also has potential as a contraceptive.

ORAL CONTRACEPTIVES

> The most common pharmacological means of preventing pregnancy is the use of estrogens and progestins to interfere with ovulation.

The mechanism of action of the oral contraceptives is not completely understood. The estrogen provides negative feedback to the pituitary, inhibiting further release of LH and FSH. This prevents ovulation. The progestin also inhibits LH and is added to stimulate withdrawal bleeding.

> Progestin alone in pill form (mini-pill) or implants also provides contraception.

The use of progestin alone is associated with irregular uterine bleeding.

> The side effects of the oral contraceptives are related to the estrogens and progestins that are part of the pills.

I hope you said "Wait, that's obvious!" The major side effects of the combination pills are breast fullness, nausea and vomiting (estrogen), depression, and edema (progestin). There is an increased incidence of abnormal clotting in women who smoke and are over the age of 35.

ANDROGENS

The androgens have masculinizing and anabolic effects in both men and women. The anabolic effects include increased muscle mass, increased bone density, and increased red blood cell mass. The virilizing effects include spermatogenesis, sexual dysfunction, or restoration and development of male characteristics. It is possible to separate (somewhat) the virilizing and anabolic activities by altering the structure of the steroid.

> TESTOSTERONE is the major androgen produced in the body.

Testosterone is produced by the Leydig cells of the testes and by the ovaries and adrenal glands. The secretion of testosterone is controlled by hormonal signals from the hypothalamus and anterior pituitary.

> The primary therapeutic use of androgens is for replacement therapy in patients with testicular deficiency.

Although the most common use of the androgens is for replacement therapy, other uses do occur. Androgens can be used to stimulate linear bone growth and in the treatment of anemia.

> The side effects of the androgens are related to their physiological actions.

This is simple enough. Androgens cause virilization of women, including acne, growth of facial hair, deepening of the voice, and excessive muscle development. In men, androgens can cause impotence, decreased spermatogenesis, gynecomastia, liver abnormalities, and psychotic episodes. In children, androgens cause closure of epiphyseal plates and abnormal sexual maturation. These should all make sense and do not need to be memorized.

ANTIANDROGENS

Competitive antagonists of testosterone include cyproterone acetate and flutamide. These drugs have been used to treat excessive hair growth in women and prostate cancer in men.

> FINASTERIDE is a 5α-reductase inhibitor that is used to treat cases of benign prostatic hypertrophy (and to stimulate hair growth).

5α-Reductase converts testosterone to dihydrotestosterone. Dihydrotestosterone is the major intracellular androgen in most target tissues. Finasteride and dutasteride (notice the similar names) are effective in slowing the growth of prostate tissue without interfering with libido (mediated by testosterone).

GnRH AGONISTS AND ANTAGONISTS

Under physiological conditions, the hypothalamus releases GnRH (also called LH-RH, see Figures 37-1) in a pulsatile manner. The frequency of the pulses controls the release of LH and FSH by the anterior pituitary.

> The hypothalamic-pituitary-gonadal axis can be suppressed by administration of either a GnRH agonist or an antagonist.

At first this doesn't make sense, but remember that GnRH release is pulsatile. Continuous administration of a GnRH agonist will suppress release of LH and FSH by desensitizing the pituitary to the activity of GnRH. The GnRH agonists, which (almost) all end in "relin," can be used in prostate cancer, endometriosis, and precocious puberty because of their suppression of estrogen and testosterone levels.

GnRH Agonists and Analogs	GnRH Antagonists
triptorelin	abarelix
nafarelin	cetrorelix
goserelin	degarelix
histrelin	ganirelix
leuprolide	

The GnRH antagonists (the "relix"s) competitively block GnRH receptors in the pituitary without causing receptor desensitization. This results in suppression of LH and FSH secretion from the anterior pituitary. Cetrorelix and ganirelix are used to inhibit premature LH surges in women undergoing fertility treatments. Abarelix is used in advanced prostate cancer.

PDE5 INHIBITORS

No, these drugs are not sex steroids, but there was no good place in the book to put it. Short of making a chapter just for one class, this seemed like as good a place as any to discuss it. These drugs are orally active agents used in the treatment of erectile dysfunction.

> Sildenafil, tadalafil, and vardenafil inhibit a phosphodiesterase found in vascular smooth muscle.

Nitric oxide is released from nerve endings and endothelial cells. It binds to receptors on the smooth muscle of the corpus cavernosum and triggers the formation of cyclic guanosine monophosphate (cGMP). cGMP causes relaxation of smooth muscle, allowing engorgement. This process is reversed by a phosphodiesterase (number 5) that converts the cGMP to GMP. Sildenafil, tadalafil, and vardenafil inhibit this phosphodiesterase.

All of these drugs potentiate the hypotensive action of nitrates. Their use together with nitrates could result in a fatal drop in blood pressure. Interestingly, sildenafil and tadalafil are also approved for the treatment of pulmonary arterial hypertension.

38

Thyroid and Parathyroid Drugs

Organization of Class
Thyroid Replacement Therapy
Drugs That Are Thyroid Downers
Parathyroid drugs

ORGANIZATION OF CLASS

These drugs are really quite simple if you can recognize the names and if you remember how the thyroid gland is controlled and how it synthesizes thyroid hormone (Figure 38–1).

The thyroid gland helps maintain an adequate level of metabolism in tissues. Hypothyroidism (low levels of hormone) results in slow heart rate (bradycardia), cold intolerance, and physical slowing. In children, hypothyroidism can result in mental retardation and short stature. Hyperthyroidism (too much hormone) results in fast heart rate, nervousness, tremor, and excess heat production.

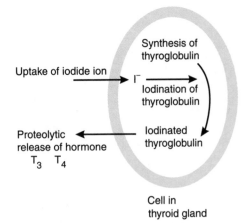

FIGURE 38–1 In each thyroid cell there is active uptake of iodide. This iodide is then incorporated onto tyrosine residues in the protein thyroglobulin. The iodinated thyroglobulin then undergoes proteolysis to release thyroid hormone in the form of T_3 and T_4.

The thyroid gland stores thyroid hormone as thyroglobulin.

THYROID REPLACEMENT THERAPY

> There are two major thyroid hormones, called T_3 and T_4. T_3 is the most active form.

T_4 is the major secretory product of the thyroid gland. T_3 is secreted by the thyroid, but is also synthesized by extrathyroid metabolism of T_4. Both T_4 and T_3 are bound to thyroxine-binding globulin and several other proteins in the plasma. T_4 is often referred to as thyroxine and T_3 as triiodothyronine.

> LEVOTHYROXINE (a sodium salt of T_4) is the most commonly used drug for thyroid replacement therapy. LEVOTHYROXINE is the *drug of choice* for the treatment of hypothyroidism.

Liothyronine (a sodium salt of T_3) and liotrix (a mixture of T_3 and T_4) have also been used to treat hypothyroidism.

DRUGS THAT ARE THYROID DOWNERS

Treatment of hyperthyroidism is achieved by removing part, or all, of the thyroid gland, inhibiting synthesis of thyroid hormone, or by blocking release of hormone from the gland.

> Surgery or radioactive iodine can be used to destroy the thyroid gland.

Remember that iodine is taken up selectively by the thyroid gland. Therefore, administration of radioactive iodine will result in the accumulation of radioactivity in the thyroid gland. This is very selective radiation therapy.

> PROPYLTHIOURACIL and METHIMAZOLE inhibit thyroid synthesis.

Propylthiouracil and methimazole inhibit iodination of tyrosine groups and coupling of these groups to form thyroid hormone. They have no effect on the stored thyroglobulin or on the release of thyroid hormone. Therefore, there will be a delay between the onset of therapy and the clinical effect as the previously stored thyroglobulin is released. Propylthiouracil also inhibits the peripheral conversion of T_4 to T_3. Propylthiouracil causes severe hepatic toxicity and is the third leading cause of liver transplants due to drug toxicity.

Note that methimazole ends in—azole, but it is NOT an antifungal agent.

PARATHYROID DRUGS

The most important endocrine regulator of calcium homeostasis is parathyroid hormone (PTH), which is secreted by the parathyroid gland.

> High serum calcium suppresses PTH secretion and low serum calcium stimulates PTH release.

PTH acts directly on the kidney to increase calcium reabsorption and on the bone to increase bone mass, while acting indirectly on the gastrointestinal (GI) tract to improve calcium absorption.

> Teriparatide is a recombinant parathyroid hormone used in the treatment of osteoporosis.

In addition to being effective in osteoporosis, teriparatide is an effective treatment for patients with hypoparathyroidism.

Hyperparathyroidism is commonly treated with synthetic vitamin D analog, such as paricalcitol and doxercalciferol.

> Cinacalet increases the sensitivity of calcium-sensing receptors in the parathyroid gland resulting in a decrease in PTH and serum calcium levels.

Cinacalet is one of a new class of drugs called calcimimetics. It can be used in the management of secondary hyperparathyroidism in patients with chronic renal failure on dialysis and in the treatment of hypercalcemia due to a parathyroid tumor.

Insulin, Glucagon, and Oral Hypoglycemic Drugs

Organization of Class
Insulins
Oral Hypoglycemic Agents

ORGANIZATION OF CLASS

A high level of glucose stimulates an increase in insulin release from β cells of the pancreas. Insulin then drives carbohydrate into cells. Patients who have high glucose levels in their blood are said to have diabetes mellitus.

Of course, you remember that diabetes mellitus is divided into two groups: type I (insulin dependent) and type II (non–insulin dependent). These distinctions are important for pharmacology because they make it easier to remember the mechanism of action of the drugs used to treat diabetes mellitus.

As an aside, there is another form of diabetes that students sometimes confuse with diabetes mellitus and that is diabetes insipidus. Diabetes insipidus is a disorder of water and sodium balance. Generally, if someone says *diabetes,* they mean the sugar-related (mellitus) disease and not diabetes insipidus.

But let's return to the topic at hand.

> Type I diabetes is related to loss of insulin-secreting cells in the pancreas. Type II diabetes is related to target cell resistance to the action of insulin.

This, of course, is somewhat simplified. An endocrinologist would cringe. Patients with type I diabetes are dependent on an exogenous (outside the body) source of insulin. This disorder generally appears in childhood; hence the former term for it is juvenile diabetes. Type II diabetes has been called adult-onset. It appears to have a genetic basis, and patients are often obese. Patients with type II diabetes are treated with oral agents that lower blood glucose (hypoglycemics) and with insulin.

So, that said, we should organize our drugs into insulins and the oral hypoglycemic agents.

INSULINS

Insulin is a small protein that is synthesized and secreted by the β cells of the pancreas. Insulin for replacement therapy can be isolated from animal sources. Human insulin is made using recombinant DNA technology.

> INSULIN must be administered by injection.

All peptides are degraded by enzymes in the gastrointestinal (GI) tract, so it is not possible to administer insulin by the oral route. Given intravenously, it has a half-life of less than 10 minutes (short). Therefore, it is administered subcutaneously.

> The most common adverse effect of insulin is hypoglycemia.

I hope that this is intuitively obvious.

> Insulin preparations vary in their time to onset and duration of action.

The onset and duration of action of the insulin preparations are controlled by the size and composition of the crystals in the particular insulin preparation.

Types of Insulin Preparations

Rapid onset and short duration

    aspart

    lispro

    insulin glulisine

    crystalline zinc insulin (regular)

    prompt insulin (SEMILENTE)

Intermediate onset and duration

    isophane insulin (NPH)

    insulin zinc (LENTE, mixture of semilente and ultralente)

Prolonged duration

    protamine zinc insulin

    extended insulin zinc (ULTRALENTE)

    insulin detemir

    insulin glargine

Basically, insulin is crystallized as a zinc salt. That's where the zinc comes from. When zinc is added to the solution, the molecules of insulin associate. These larger molecules diffuse more slowly. The rapidly acting analogues, lispro and aspart, are formulated to dissociate rapidly. The protamine is a positively charged peptide mixture that delays the absorption of the insulin (less soluble complex). In other words, reducing the solubility decreases the absorption and increases the duration of action. Insulin detemir reversibly binds to albumin, which increases its duration of action. Just as an aside, NPH stands for neutral protamine Hagedorn.

ORAL HYPOGLYCEMIC AGENTS

The oral hypoglycemic agents are so named because they lower blood glucose (hypoglycemic) and can be administered orally (as opposed to insulin). That makes the route of administration easy to remember. These drugs are organized in different ways by different textbooks. Look and see how your book or class organizes them.

Oral Hypoglycemic Agents

Sulfonylureas	*Thiazolidinediones (TZDs)*
glimepiride	rosiglitazone
glipizide	pioglitazone
glyburide	*Others*
non–sulfonylureas secretagogues	metformin—biguanide
nateglinide	sitagliptin—DDP-4 inhibitor
repaglinide	exenatide—GLP-1 receptor agonist
α-Glucosidase inhibitors	liraglutide—GLP-1 receptor agonist
acarbose	pramlintide—amylin analogue
miglitol	colesevelam—bile acid sequestrant

> The sulfonylureas act by stimulating the release of insulin from the β cells in the pancreas by an interaction with the ATP-sensitive potassium channels.

The sulfonylureas stimulate insulin release, reduce serum glucagon levels, and increase binding of insulin to target tissues. The "glinides"(nateglinide and repaglinide) also stimulate release of insulin from the pancreas. Historically, the sulfonylureas were divided into two groups: first generation and second generation. The first-generation durgs are rarely used anymore having been replaced by the second-generation drugs. The drugs vary in their duration of action and side effects. For now, name recognition is the most important thing for you to focus on.

Repaglinide and nateglinide also bind to the ATP-sensitive potassium channels on the β cells to increase insulin release, but are not structurally sulfonylureas, hence the categorization as non–sulfonylureas secretagogues.

> The most common adverse effect of the sulfonylureas is hypoglycemia.

I hope you can remember that without too much problem.

The α-glucosidase inhibitors (acarbose and miglitol) are nicknamed the "starch blockers". They increase the time required for absorption of carbohydrates, thus reducing the peak glucose levels after eating. They will not reduce hyperglycemia at other times.

> The "glitazones" increase sensitivity to insulin.

The "glitazones" are thiazolidinediones (TZDs). These drugs enhance the action of insulin at target tissues by acting as agonists for the nuclear hormone receptor called peroxisome proliferator activated receptor-gamma (PPAR-γ). PPAR-γ regulates the production of proteins involved in glucose and lipid metabolism. There is on-going concern about possible increased risk of heart attacks in patients on these drugs.

> Metformin also increases insulin sensitivity. A rare, but potentially fatal, side effect is lactic acidosis, particularly in patients with renal impairment.

Metformin is considered a "biguanide." It decreases glucose output from the liver and increases peripheral glucose utilization.

Sitagliptin is what's called a dipeptidyl-peptidase-4 (DPP-4) inhibitor. DPP-4 is responsible for inactivation and degradation of two GI hormones that lower serum glucose production, GLP-1 and glucose-dependent insulinotropic polypeptide (GIP). These GI hormones potentiate insulin synthesis and release by β cells in the pancreas and decrease glucagon production by α cells. When you inhibit the degradation of these hormones, they can continue to lower serum glucose.

> Exenatide, liraglutide, and pramlintide are peptides that lower serum glucose levels, slow gastric emptying, and increase satiety.

Exenatide and liraglutide are peptides similar to the incretin hormone glucagon-like peptide-1 (GLP-1), which in the presence of glucose acts to stimulate insulin secretion. Pramlintide is a synthetic analogue of amylin, a small peptide hormone that is released into the bloodstream by the β cells of the pancreas along with insulin. Amylin reduces the production of glucose by the liver by inhibiting the action of glucagon.

CHAPTER 40:   Histamine and Antihistamines   205

CHAPTER 41:   Respiratory Drugs   208

CHAPTER 42:   Drugs That Affect the GI Tract   212

CHAPTER 43:   Nonnarcotic Analgesics and Anti-inflammatory Drugs   216

CHAPTER 44:   Immunosuppressives   223

CHAPTER 45:   Drugs Used in Osteoporosis   225

CHAPTER 46:   Toxicology and Poisoning   228

Histamine and Antihistamines

Organization of Class
H_1 Receptor Antagonists

ORGANIZATION OF CLASS

Histamine is an endogenous substance that is widely distributed throughout the body. The two principal sites of storage for histamine are the mast cells in tissue and the basophils in blood.

> The action of histamine is mediated through at least two receptors, H_1 and H_2.

H_3 receptors have been reported in the brain, but for our purposes there are two classes of histamine receptors.

> Intestinal and bronchial smooth muscles contain mostly H_1 receptors. Gastric secretion is mediated by H_2 receptors.

As you can see, the action of histamine depends on the receptors with which it interacts. Histamine itself, or agonists of the histamine receptors, have only minor uses in clinical medicine. Because we consider drugs that act on the GI tract in the following chapter, we will not consider the H_2 receptor antagonists any further here.

H_1 RECEPTOR ANTAGONISTS

H_1 Receptor Antagonists	
DIPHENHYDRAMINE	chlorpheniramine
acrivastine	dimenhydrinate
azelastine	hydroxyzine
brompheniramine	meclizine

(Continued)

clemastine	promethazine
cyclizine	
cyproheptadine	
olopatadine	
Nonsedating Antihistamines	
astemizole	
cetirizine	
desloratadine	
fexofenadine	
levocetirizine	
loratadine	

As always, compare this list with the one in your textbook or class handouts and make any adjustments. Some books will divide these drugs into first generation and second generation H_1 antihistamines, or into sedating versus nonsedating groups. Second-generation antihistamines do not cross into the brain as easily as the first-generation drugs and are, therefore, less likely to have CNS side effects. Because many of the first-generation drugs are available over the counter, they are more recognizable by their trade names. They are inexpensive, but have significant side effects, including sedation and anticholinergic effects.

> These drugs are competitive antagonists of the H_1 receptor.

> The H_1 antagonists (antihistamines) are used to treat cases of allergic rhinitis and motion sickness, and sometimes to induce sleep.

First, note that this class of drugs is commonly referred as antihistamines. This is in spite of the fact that there is a whole group of H_2 antagonists that could also be called antihistamines, but aren't.

The most common use of antihistamines is in the treatment of runny nose caused by seasonal allergies. The first-generation drugs cross the blood–brain barrier. In the CNS, they interact with histamine receptors and cause sedation. This effect is sometimes used therapeutically. A number of these drugs are used to treat motion sickness (diphenhydramine, dimenhydrinate, cyclizine, and meclizine). This action may be the result of a central antihistamine effect or a central anticholinergic action. The various agents in this class vary in terms of their anticholinergic potency, the degree of sedation they induce, and their duration of action.

The nonsedating antihistamines, that is, the ones belonging to second generation (astemizole, cetirizine, fexofenadine, desloratidine, and loratadine) do not cross the blood–brain barrier, so are less sedating.

Be absolutely sure you know the names of these second-generation nonsedating antihistamines. These are first-line therapy for mild to moderate allergic rhinitis. The first nonsedating antihistamine, terfenadine, has been removed from the market.

41 Respiratory Drugs

Organization of Class
β-Agonists
Leukotriene Modifiers
Methylxanthines
Cholinergic Antagonists
Cromolyn and Omalizumab
Pulmonary Hypertension

ORGANIZATION OF CLASS

Bronchoconstriction, inflammation, and loss of lung elasticity are the most common processes that result in respiratory compromise. Bronchoconstriction can be treated with adrenergic agonists, cholinergic antagonists, and some other compounds. Inflammation is treatable with corticosteroids. Obstruction of the airways can also occur with infection and increased secretions. The infection is treated with antibiotics. Because the antibiotics and steroids have been covered elsewhere, this chapter focuses on the bronchodilators. Most of this will be a review from autonomics.

> Drugs used in the treatment of bronchoconstriction include inhaled corticosteroids, β-agonists, cholinergic antagonists, and methylxanthines.

If you add cromolyn and the leukotriene modifiers, which are prophylactic agents, and corticosteroids for chronic treatment, you are all set.

Most of these drugs are now administered by inhalation. This gets the drug to the site of action and should limit the systemic effects.

> β_2-Agonists cause bronchodilation.

Inhaled corticosteroids used in the treatment of asthma include:

beclomethasone	fluticasone
budesonide	mometasone
ciclesonide	triamcinolone
flunisolide	

β-AGONISTS

Inhaled short-acting β_2-agonists are the most effective drugs available for treatment of acute bronchospasm and for prevention of exercise-induced asthma. β_2-Selective agents are preferred, to avoid the cardiac effect of β_1-activation. Use of long-acting β_2-agonists has been associated with an increased risk of asthma-related death, intubation or hospitalization, and it is no longer recommended that long-acting β_2-agonists be used as monotherapy for asthma.

There are a number of β-agonists that are used in the treatment of asthma and chronic obstructive pulmonary disease (COPD).

β-Agonists Used As Bronchodilators

ALBUTEROL (SA)	arformoterol (LA)
levalbuterol (SA)	formoterol (LA)
pirbuterol (SA)	salmeterol (LA)
SA, short-acting; LA, long acting	

In an emergency, such as the bronchoconstriction associated with anaphylaxis, epinephrine can be used. Use of a short-acting β-agonist more than two to three times a week means that the asthma is not well controlled and adjustments to baseline medication need to be made. Long-acting β-agonists can be used in combination with inhaled corticosteroids to control asthma symptoms.

LEUKOTRIENE MODIFIERS

Leukotriene modifiers can be used as an alternative to inhaled corticosteroids, but they are less effective. Cysteinyl leukotrienes are products of arachidonic acid metabolism. They increase eosinophil migration, mucus production, and airway wall edema, and cause bronchoconstriction. Montelukast and zafirlukast block binding of LTD_4 (the predominant cysteinyl leukotriene in the airways) to its receptor. Zileuton inhibits leukotriene synthesis by inhibiting 5-lipoxygenase, which catalyzes the conversion of arachidonic acid to leukotrienes.

Leukotriene modifiers are approved for oral prophylaxis and chronic treatment of asthma.

Leukotriene modifiers are not recommended for treatment of an acute asthma attack.

METHYLXANTHINES

Theophylline (or aminophylline) was once the treatment of choice for the management of asthma. The primary drugs are now the inhaled corticosteroids and β_2-agonists. The methyl-xanthines increase cAMP levels, but the exact mechanism by which they cause bronchodilation is not known. Theophylline is still listed as a treatment option for COPD. It is rare that students mistake these drugs for another class of compounds. The ending "-phylline" is a dead giveaway.

CHOLINERGIC ANTAGONISTS

The cholinergic antagonists block the bronchoconstriction caused by activation of the parasympathetic nervous system.

> IPRATROPIUM (short-acting) and tiotropium (long-acting) are anticholinergic agents used for the treatment of COPD in adults.

The cholinergic antagonist, ipratropium, has found use in the treatment of chronic obstructive pulmonary disease (COPD). Ipratropium is less effective against asthma.

CROMOLYN AND OMALIZUMAB

> CROMOLYN sodium is used prophylactically in the treatment of asthma.

Cromolyn is *not* useful in the treatment of an acute attack and is infrequently used these days. The mechanism of action of cromolyn is not clear. It does block the release of mediators from mast cells, but the relevance of this action has been questioned.

> Omalizumab is a monoclonal antibody specific for IgE and is used for the treatment of allergic asthma.

You should already know that omalizumab is a monoclonal antibody because the name ends in "mab." It binds to IgE's high-affinity Fc receptor, lowering the serum concentration of free IgE and preventing binding of IgE to a variety of cells, including mast cells. This will prevent activation (and degranulation) of these cells. As opposed to cromolyn, omalizumab will also reduce the late phase of the allergic response by preventing IgE binding to other cells throughout the body.

PULMONARY HYPERTENSION

Pulmonary arterial hypertension (PAH) is an uncommon disease characterized by increased pulmonary artery pressure and vascular resistance. The predominant symptom is shortness of breath—hence it's inclusion in the chapter on respiratory drugs. Data indicate that inflammation has a prominent role in the pathogenesis of PAH. Also, endothelin-1 levels are increased in plasma and lung tissue of patients with PAH, suggesting a role of endothelin-1 in the pathogenesis.

> Endothelin-receptor antagonists (ambrisentan and bosentan) and prostocyclin analogs (epoprostenol, iloprost, and treprostinil) are available for use in pulmonary hypertension.

Bosentan is a specific and competitive antagonist of both type A and B endothelin-1 receptors, while ambrisentan is specific for type A receptors. Both can improve exercise ability and slow the progression of the disease. Bosentan lowers systemic vascular resistance, pulmonary vascular resistance, and mean pulmonary arterial pressure. Both of these drugs can be given orally. The PDE5 inhibitors, sildenafil and tadalafil, can also be used for PAH.

The prostacyclin analogues are reserved for more advanced disease, in part because they must be given by injection.

CHAPTER 42

Drugs That Affect the GI Tract

Organization of Class
Drugs That Act in the Upper GI Tract
Drugs That Act in the Lower GI Tract

ORGANIZATION OF CLASS

The organization of these drugs is based on the organization of the GI tract. There are drugs that are used in treating ulcers in the stomach and duodenum. There are also drugs that affect motility in the upper GI tract. Then, moving down to the large intestine, we can divide the agents into those that enhance motility and those that reduce motility. Finally, there are agents that specifically target diseases of the lower GI tract.

DRUGS THAT ACT IN THE UPPER GI TRACT

Duodenal and gastric ulcers are often caused by the bacterium *Helicobacter pylori*. The treatment objective is eradication of *H. pylori* with a combination of antibiotics and H_2 blockers. Bismuth (PEPTO-BISMOL) appears to be bactericidal to *H. pylori*.

> The "proton pump inhibitors" (the "..prazoles") inhibit the H^+-K^+-ATPase enzyme of the parietal cell. This reduces acid secretion.
> OMEPRAZOLE
> ESOMEPRAZOLE
> deslansoprazole (delayed-release formulation of the R-enantionmer of lansoprazole)
> lansoprazole
> pantoprazole
> rabeprazole

These drugs are superior to H_2 antagonists in the suppression of acid and in the healing of peptic ulcers.

H$_2$ receptor antagonists prevent histamine-induced acid release. H$_2$ antagonists include:
CIMETIDINE—watch out for drug interactions!
RANITIDINE
famotidine
nizatidine

These drugs are easily recognizable by the "-tidine" ending. These drugs are used for the short-term treatment of gastroesophageal reflux and peptic ulcer disease. Cimetidine binds to cytochrome P-450. Therefore, adverse drug interactions with drugs transformed via the cytochrome P-450 system are common with cimetidine.

The aluminum salts and calcium carbonate antacids cause constipation. The magnesium salts cause diarrhea. Therefore, they are often mixed.

Antacids can decrease the absorption of other drugs because they alter the stomach and duodenal pH. They can also bind to drugs and block their absorption. This is particularly true for the aluminum salts. Antacids also have systemic effects. Magnesium salts can cause hypermagnesemia and aluminum salts can cause hypophosphatemia.

SUCRALFATE forms a protective coating on the mucosa, particularly ulcerated areas.

Sucralfate is only minimally absorbed. Constipation is the main side effect.

Metoclopramide and cisapride increase the rate of gastric emptying.

Metoclopramide has both peripheral and central effects. Centrally, it is a dopamine antagonist and has produced extrapyramidal side effects. Peripherally, it stimulates release of acetylcholine. Cisapride has been removed from the market in the United States due to cardiac arrhythmias.

MISOPROSTOL is a prostaglandin analogue that increases bicarbonate and mucin release and reduces acid secretion. It is used to treat NSAID-induced ulceration.

DRUGS THAT ACT IN THE LOWER GI TRACT

Diarrhea is most often caused by infection, toxins, or drugs. Bacterial or parasitic diarrhea should be treated with the appropriate agent for the infection. Drug-induced diarrhea should be treated by discontinuation of the drug, if possible. An example of targeted therapy for diarrhea is the use of octreotide (synthetic somatostatin) for the diarrhea associated with vasoactive intestinal peptide secreting tumors and metastatic carcinoid tumors (they secrete serotonin).

Opiates that are used to treat diarrhea include DIPHENOXYLATE and LOPERAMIDE. These should *not* be used for an infectious process. There are also absorbent powders such as KAOPECTATE that are used in the treatment of diarrhea. Bismuth subsalicylate (PEPTO-BISMOL) may coat irritated mucosal surfaces.

Drugs used to treat constipation can be divided into two groups: the bulk-forming agents and the stimulants and cathartics. These drugs are also taken orally. Some can be administered by insertion into the rectum.

The bulk-forming agents used to treat constipation contain plant matter that absorbs water and softens the stool. These include:
calcium polycarbophil
methylcellulose
psyllium

The stimulants used to treat constipation increase water and electrolytes in the feces and increase motility. These include:
bisacodyl
danthron
phenolphthalein
senna

You probably recognize these more by their trade names of METAMUCIL (psyllium), DULCOLAX (bisacodyl), and EX LAX (phenolphthalein). It helps to remember which are bulk-formers and which are stimulants.

There are a couple of others that you may be asked about. Saline salts of magnesium and sodium (MILK OF MAGNESIA) draw water into the colon. Docusate (COLACE) improves penetration of water and fat into feces.

Lubiprostone, a prostaglandin E1 analog, is approved for the treatment of chronic constipation and irritable bowel syndrome with constipation. It activates chloride channels in the epithelium of the GI tract, stimulating intestinal fluid secretion.

5-Aminosalicylate (5-ASA) is the active metabolite of SULFASALAZINE, which is used to treat inflammatory bowel disease.

The primary therapy for inflammatory bowel disease (ulcerative colitis and Crohn's disease) utilizes steroids and 5-aminosalicyclate (5-ASA), also called mesalamine, to control the inflammatory process. 5-ASA probably inhibits leukotriene production and has antiprostaglandin and antioxidant activity. Sulfasalazine, balsalazide and olsalazine (prodrugs for mesalamine), and mesalamine itself are used in mild to moderate ulcerative colitis and for maintenance of remission in ulcerative colitis.

Other immunomodulating agents are also used in inflammatory bowel disease, including azathioprine, mercaptopurine, methotrexate, and cyclosporine

(Chaps 35 and 44). In addition, antibodies and antibody fragments that bind to tumor necrosis factor alpha (TNF-α) block the inflammatory cascade and can be used in inflammatory bowel disease. Infliximab and adalimumab are monoclonal antibodies that bind to and inhibit TNF-α. Certolizumab pegol is an antibody fragment that is also used. These TNF-α inhibitors are general reserved for disease refractory to more conventional therapy. Natalizumab is another monoclonal antibody that is used in Crohn's disease. It reduces intestinal inflammation by binding α-4 integrin, a molecule that mediates adhesion of leukocytes to endothelial receptors.

For irritable bowel syndrome in women, alosetron has shown some efficacy, but also very serious side effects. It is a 5-HT$_3$ receptor antagonist.

> Orlistat is a lipase inhibitor being used to treat obesity.

Orlistat binds to pancreatic and gastric lipase and inactivates the enzyme. This reduces the absorption of dietary fat by about 30%. Adverse effects include flatulence, oily spotting, and fecal urgency.

43

Nonnarcotic Analgesics and Anti-inflammatory Drugs

Organization of Class

Nonsteroidal Anti-inflammatory Drugs (NSAIDs)

COX-2 Inhibitors

Salicylates, Including Aspirin

Acetaminophen

Other Drugs for Arthritis

Antigout Agents

Drugs Used in the Treatment of Headaches

ORGANIZATION OF CLASS

Some textbooks put these drugs after the opiate analgesics and others group the antiarthritis drugs together. Basically we will consider here some salient features of the nonnarcotic analgesics and some of the anti-inflammatory agents. I've also included the drugs used for gout and migraines. The largest group of drugs here is the nonsteroidal anti-inflammatory drugs (NSAIDs). This group includes aspirin and the salicylates. However, the salicylates and aspirin have some important special features, so I have separated them to emphasize these features.

NONSTEROIDAL ANTI-INFLAMMATORY DRUGS

NSAIDs

IBUPROFEN	meclofenamate
INDOMETHACIN	nabumetone
KETOROLAC	oxaprozin
NAPROXEN	phenylbutazone
diclofenac	piroxicam
etodolac	sulindac

(Continued)

NSAIDs (*Continued*)

fenoprofen	suprofen
flurbiprofen	tolmetin
ketoprofen	
meloxicam	
mefenamic acid	

Compare this list with the one in your textbook or class handouts. There seems to be no rhyme or reason to the names.

> *All* the NSAIDs (including aspirin) are thought to exert their clinical effects by inhibiting prostaglandin synthesis.

The primary site of action is the cyclooxygenase (COX) enzyme, which catalyzes the conversion of arachidonic acid to prostaglandin and endoperoxide (Figure 43–1). Prostaglandins modulate components of inflammation. They also are involved in control of body temperature, pain transmission, platelet aggregation, and other effects. They are not stored by cells, but are synthesized and released on demand. Their half-lives are only minutes long. Therefore, if you control the enzyme that makes prostaglandins, then you control the prostaglandins themselves.

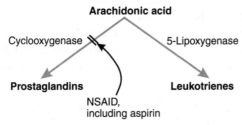

FIGURE 43–1 Remember that arachidonic acid is converted to both prostaglandins and leukotrienes. The NSAIDs inhibit the enzyme cyclooxygenase and, therefore, the formation of prostaglandins.

> *All* the NSAIDs (including aspirin) have analgesic, antipyretic, and anti-inflammatory effects. The older (nonspecific) NSAIDs also have antithrombotic effects.

The NSAIDs (including aspirin) are used in the treatment of moderate pain, fever, tendinitis, sunburn, rheumatoid arthritis, and osteoarthritis, just to name a few.

> The most common adverse effects of the NSAIDs (including aspirin) are GI injury and renal injury.

GI injury consists of gastritis and ulcers. Misoprostol, a synthetic prostaglandin analogue, is used for the prevention of NSAID-induced ulcers. NSAIDs can cause oliguria, fluid retention, decreased sodium excretion, renal failure, and can prolong bleeding time.

The agents differ with respect to their CNS side effects, duration of action, degree of platelet antagonism (bleeding), and GI toxicity.

> KETOROLAC is an NSAID that can be administered intramuscularly or intravenously. Ibuprofen is now also available for intravenous administration.

COX-2 INHIBITORS

Two isoforms of the COX enzyme have been identified. COX-1 is expressed constitutively in most tissues and is thought to protect the gastric mucosa. COX-2 is expressed constitutively in brain and kidney and is induced at sites of inflammation. COX-1, but not COX-2, is present in platelets. The older NSAIDs block both COX isoforms. Theoretically, a specific COX-2 inhibitor should be anti-inflammatory without harming the GI tract or altering platelet function.

COX-2 inhibitors are all named with the ending "coxib." They include celecoxib, etoricoxib, rofecoxib, and valdecoxib.

In 2004, a study was released that showed an increase in the risk of cardiovascular disease in patients taking COX-2 inhibitors. In response to this study, rofecoxib and valdecoxib were withdrawn from the market in the United States. There is ongoing debate about the relative safety of these drugs versus the potential benefits. The increased risk of cardiovascular disease is thought to be related to a decrease in the formation of PGI_2. PGI_2 inhibits platelet aggregation and prevents proliferation of vascular smooth muscle in vitro and causes vasodilation.

SALICYLATES, INCLUDING ASPIRIN

> Aspirin causes irreversible inactivation of COX. It is the only NSAID to do this.

Aspirin, and other salicylates, are metabolized to salicylic acid, which is the active agent (Figure 43–2). Aspirin acetylates the COX enzyme, causing irreversible inactivation of the enzyme. Therefore, its effect lasts until the body makes more enzyme.

Aspirin brings down a fever, reduces minor pain, reduces inflammation, and prevents blood clots. The antipyretic and analgesic actions are mediated by an action in the CNS. Aspirin has been shown to prevent heart attacks, probably due to its anticlotting action via inhibition of the production of thromboxane A_2.

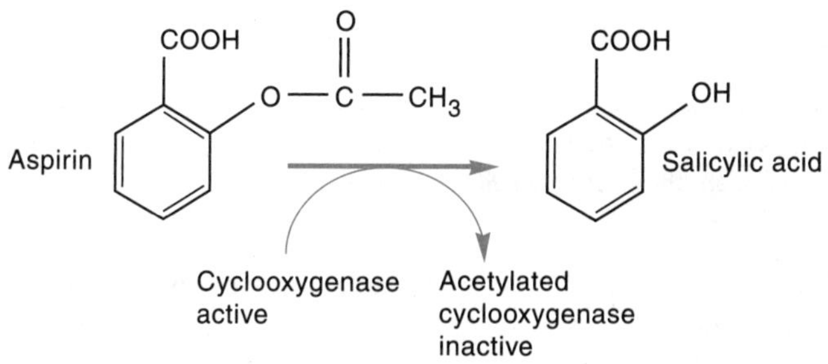

FIGURE 43–2 Aspirin is metabolized to salicylic acid by the removal of the acetate group. If the acetate is taken by the cyclooxygenase enzyme, then the enzyme is inactivated. In this way aspirin causes an irreversible inhibition of cyclooxygenase.

Aspirin is now also considered an essential element in the management of an acute myocardial infarction.

> Use of aspirin has been associated with Reye syndrome in children.

Reye syndrome is characterized by CNS damage, liver injury, and hypoglycemia. Its cause is unknown. The incidence of Reye syndrome has fallen dramatically with education of the public not to give aspirin to children.

> Overdose of aspirin is called salicylism. Symptoms include ringing in the ears (tinnitus), dizziness, headache, fever, and mental status changes.

Notice that overdose can cause the very symptoms that the patient set out to treat (headache, fever).

> The pH changes after ingestion of large amounts of aspirin are complex, but important to understand.
> 1. Stimulation of the medullary respiratory center causes an increase in ventilation. This leads to *respiratory alkalosis* ($\uparrow$pH and $\downarrow$pCO$_2$).
> 2. There is uncoupling of oxidative phosphorylation. This leads to an increase in plasma CO$_2$, which further stimulates the respiratory center.

> Aspirin has zero-order kinetics.

Remember zero-order kinetics? Aspirin and salicylic acid are metabolized by glucuronidation—an enzymatic reaction that can be saturated. Therefore, elimination can become zero-order (saturation kinetics). This is reflected in the plasma half-life, which increases with increasing doses. Remember that aspirin has a very long duration of action because of the irreversible inactivation of COX. This is another example of the half-life not matching the duration of action.

ACETAMINOPHEN

> ACETAMINOPHEN has analgesic and antipyretic actions, but does *not* have anti-inflammatory or antithrombotic activity.

Acetaminophen only weakly inhibits prostaglandin synthesis and has no effect on platelet aggregation.

> ACETAMINOPHEN can cause *fatal* liver damage.

In overdose, the major concern is liver damage. This is apparently mediated by the binding of a toxic metabolite to the liver itself (Figure 43–3). Toxicity can be prevented by IV administration of sulfhydryl donors such as *N*-acetylcysteine, if treatment is initiated quickly.

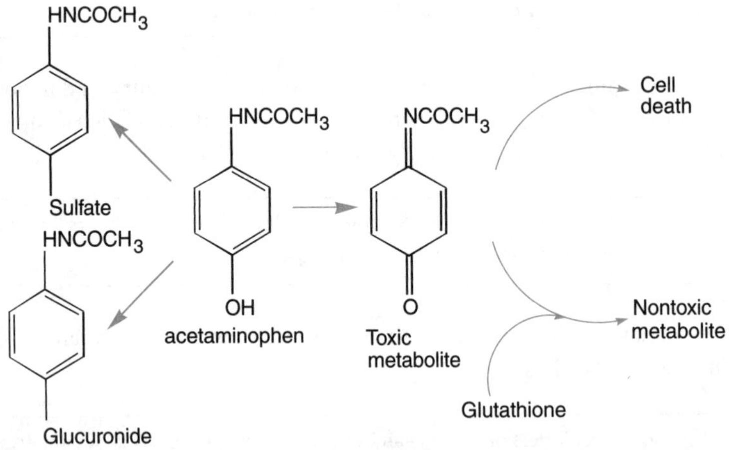

FIGURE 43–3 Acetaminophen can be metabolized in three directions (*arrows*). One direction gives a metabolite that is toxic to liver cells. However, glutathione can bind to the toxic metabolite and make it nontoxic. There are only limited quantities of glutathione available. Therefore, high doses of acetaminophen can be toxic.

OTHER DRUGS FOR ARTHRITIS

Disease-modifying antirheumatic drugs (DMARDs) are used early in the treatment of rheumatoid arthritis to prevent irreversible damage. Methotrexate (Chapter 35), an antifolate, is usually the DMARD of choice. Leflunomide is an inhibitor of pyrimidine synthesis that also can be used as initial therapy. Other nonbiologic DMARDs include the immunosuppressants azathioprine, cyclosporine, and sulfasalazine.

> Some gold preparations are used in the treatment of rheumatoid arthritis.

Auranofin is an orally effective gold preparation.

The other commonly used gold preparations are aurothioglucose and gold sodium thiomalate. If you remember that Au stands for gold on the periodic table (general chemistry, remember?), then you should not have a problem with name recognition. The mechanism of action of these compounds is not known. The most important thing here is to recognize the names.

Adalimumab, etanercept, and infliximab, inhibitors of tumor necrosis factor activity, can be used in the treatment of rheumatoid arthritis.

These drugs are considered biologic DMARDs. Adalimu*mab*, inflixi*mab*, and golimu*mab*, obviously monoclonal antibodies, bind to tumor necrosis factor-α (TNF-α) and block the interaction of TNF-α with its receptors. Etanercept inhibits TNF-α by binding to and inactivating it. Remember that TNF-α is a naturally occurring cytokine that is involved in normal inflammatory and immune responses. Elevated levels of TNF-α are thought to play an important role in the inflammation and joint destruction in rheumatoid arthritis. These drugs are also used in inflammatory bowel disease (Chapter 42).

A variety of other antibodies against inflammatory molecules are now available and more are likely to appear over the next several years. Rituximab is a monoclonal antibody against CD20, a surface antigen on B cells. Abatacept is a protein that interferes with T-cell activation. Tocilizumab is an antibody to the pro-inflammatory cytokine IL-6.

Anakinra is a recombinant form of the human interleukin-1 (IL-1) receptor antagonist. It will block the effects of IL-1, which is one of the primary pro-inflammatory cytokines associated with rheumatoid arthritis. IL-1 acts synergistically with TNF-α.

ANTIGOUT AGENTS

Just a few facts here that you should be sure you know. Remember that gout is a buildup of uric acid in tissues. Inflammation is caused by migration of leukocytes to the joint in an attempt to clear away the uric acid crystals.

You need to distinguish between acute and chronic gout. For acute gout, colchicine, NSAIDs, or intra-articular glucocorticoids can be used. NSAIDs are the treatment of choice for acute flare-ups.

Colchicine can be used in acute attacks of gouty arthritis. It reduces inflammation.

Colchicine inhibits neutrophil activation. Hyperuricemia should be treated in patients with recurrent attacks, and in those with chronic gout or evidence of tophi.

ALLOPURINOL and febuxostat are urate-lowering agents that inhibit xanthine oxidase, thus reducing synthesis of uric acid.

Before starting treatment with urate-lowering agents, the patient should be free of all signs of inflammation. Pharmacological treatment of hyperuricemia attempts to increase renal excretion of uric acid by decreasing tubular reabsorption or attempts to decrease synthesis of uric acid (Figure 43–4). Probenecid can be used to increase excretion of uric acid.

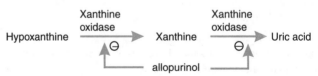

FIGURE 43–4 Uric acid is formed from hypoxanthine and xanthine by the enzyme xanthine oxidase. Allopurinol inhibits xanthine oxidase.

DRUGS USED IN THE TREATMENT OF HEADACHES

NSAIDs are the mainstay of the treatment of headaches, including migraines.

5-HT$_1$-Receptor Agonists ("-Triptans")

almotriptan	rizatriptan
eletriptan	sumatriptan
frovatriptan	ZOLMITRIPTAN
naratriptan	

The selective 5-HT$_1$-receptor agonists are highly effective for the treatment of acute migraine. They act on intracranial blood vessels and peripheral sensory nerve endings, resulting in vasoconstriction and decreased release of inflammatory neuropeptides. They appear to be more effective for treatment of acute migraine attacks than the ergot alkaloids. Injectable and nasal forms of sumatriptan have faster onset of action than oral forms.

The ergot alkaloids (dihydroergotamine and ergotamine) are most effective when taken early in an attack. If used frequently, a rebound headache can occur. These guys can have serious side effects.

A large number of compounds in a variety of drug classes have been used for prevention of migraine. None have achieved notable success. For continuous prophylaxis, β-blockers are most commonly used.

Immunosuppressives

Organization of Class
Calcineurin Inhibitors
Mycophenolate Mofetil and Azathioprine
Monoclonal Antibodies

ORGANIZATION OF CLASS

Immunopharmacology is the study of the use of drugs to modulate the immune response. The principal application of this field to clinical medicine is with drugs that suppress the immune response. These drugs are used in the treatment of autoimmune diseases (myasthenia gravis and rheumatoid arthritis) and in organ transplantation.

> Glucocorticoids
> Calcineurin inhibitors
>   CICLOSPORIN
>   tacrolimus
>   sirolimus
>   everolimus
>   pimecrolimus
> Inhibitor of nucleotide synthesis
>   mycophenolate mofetil
> Antimetabolite
>   azathioprine
> Antibodies
>   muromonab (anti-CD3)
>   daclizumab, basiliximab (anti-CD25)

CALCINEURIN INHIBITORS

> CICLOSPORINE inhibits antibody and cell-mediated immune responses and is the *drug of choice* for prevention of transplant rejection.

Ciclosporine (also cyclosporin) binds to cyclophilin (an intracellular protein of the immunophilin family), while everolimus (derivative of sirolimus), sirolimus, and tacrolimus bind to a protein called FKBP12, another immunophilin. For all of these drugs, the drug-protein complex then inhibits calcineurin phosphatase and T-cell activation. Nephrotoxicity is the major side effect of ciclosporine.

MYCOPHENOLATE MOFETIL AND AZATHIOPRINE

Mycophenolate mofetil is administered as a prodrug that is activated to mycophenolic acid—the active compound. It is a highly selective inhibitor of a crucial enzyme in the de novo synthesis of guanosine. Proliferating lymphocytes are dependent on the de novo pathway for purine biosynthesis. Most other cell lines can maintain function with the salvage pathway. Therefore, mycophenolic acid is a very specific lymphocyte inhibitor.

Azathioprine is thought to be immunosuppressive by interfering with DNA synthesis.

MONOCLONAL ANTIBODIES

Muromonab is a mouse monoclonal antibody that binds to the CD3 protein complex on T lymphocytes, blocking antigen recognition.

Basiliximab and daclizumab block the interleukin-2 (IL-2)–mediated activation of T lymphocytes by binding to CD25, which is the α chain of the interleukin-2 receptor.

Drugs Used in Osteoporosis

Organization of Class
Bisphosphonates
Selective Estrogen Receptor Modulators (SERMs)
Estrogens
Parathyroid hormone
Calcitonin
Other Agents

ORGANIZATION OF CLASS

The choices for the prevention and treatment of osteoporosis have expanded significantly in the past 5 years and probably will continue to change in the coming years. Some of these drugs have been covered elsewhere, but many of these drugs do not fit into other categories, so this chapter was created to pull this information together in one place.

Osteoporosis is the term used for a set of diseases characterized by the loss of bone mass. It is the most common of the metabolic bone diseases and is an important cause of morbidity in the elderly.

> Pharmacological therapy is targeted toward both prevention of bone loss and treatment of established osteoporosis (increasing bone mass and reducing fractures).

Remember that bone is constantly forming and resorbing. The rates of the remodeling vary between people, between different bones, and at different ages. Diet and exercise play a major role in maintenance of bone mass. Intake of calcium and vitamin D are critical and supplements have been used for the treatment of osteoporosis. Calcium is not well absorbed from the gut and vitamin D improves absorption. Vitamin D levels are now being tested and daily recommended intake has been increasing.

Calcium supplementation has been shown to reduce bone loss in postmenopausal women, but not to increase bone density once lost. Calcium supplements are available in a variety of salts.

BISPHOSPHONATES

> ALENDRONATE
> clodronate
> etidronate
> pamidronate
> risedronate
> tiludronate
> zoledronate

> The bisphosphonates inhibit osteoclastic activity and decrease bone turnover and resorption. They have been shown to reduce the incidence of fractures.

These agents have been shown to improve bone mass in established osteoporosis. They are not well absorbed from the GI tract, and absorption is decreased even more by the presence of food. They bind to bone, thus having a lasting effect from a single dose. This is the basis of the once weekly or once yearly dosing now available. The half-life of alendronate in bone has been measured to be at least 10 years.

SELECTIVE ESTROGEN RECEPTOR MODULATORS

These compounds were introduced in Chapter 37. The selective estrogen receptor modulators have different degrees of estrogen agonist or antagonist activity in different tissues.

> Raloxifene has been approved for the prevention of postmenopausal osteoporosis.

Raloxifene is an estrogen agonist on bone and an antagonist in both the breast and uterus. Raloxifene has been shown to reduce the incidence of vertebral fractures without increasing the risk of breast or uterine cancer. It is not as effective as estrogen at increasing bone density. Like estrogen, the selective estrogen receptor modulators (SERMs) can increase the risk for thromboembolism.

ESTROGENS

Estrogens were covered in more detail in Chapter 37. Estrogen can to prevent bone loss after menopause. Estrogen is not as effective at increasing bone mass that has already been lost.

PARATHYROID HORMONE

> Teriparatide, recombinant parathyroid hormone, is effective in reducing the incidence of new fractures in patients with osteoporosis.

Parathyroid hormone was reviewed in Chapter 38. Unlike other treatments for osteoporosis, teriparatide stimulates the formation of new bone and increases bone mass. It must be given by injection.

CALCITONIN

Normally produced in the body, calcitonin regulates calcium levels by inhibiting osteoclastic activity (breakdown of bone). Calcitonin can be used in established osteoporosis, but studies have not shown a clear benefit to its use. It must be administered subcutaneously or by nasal spray. Calcitonin does have some analgesic action, which may be of benefit in patients with fractures.

OTHER AGENTS

Denosumab, a monoclonal antibody (but you knew that, right?), is a RANK ligand inhibitor. RANK is "receptor activator of nuclear factor-κB." Denosumab prevents the interaction of the ligand with the receptor on cells of osteoclastic lineage. Remember that osteoclasts break down bone and activation of the RANK receptor stimulates osteoclasts. Thus blocking this receptor will inhibit bone resorption.

46 Toxicology and Poisoning

Principles of Toxicology
General Principles in the Treatment of Poisoning
Specific Antidotes

PRINCIPLES OF TOXICOLOGY

Toxicology is the study of the toxic or harmful effects of chemicals. It is also concerned with the symptoms and treatment of poisoning and the identification of the poison.

The variety of potential adverse effects and the diversity of chemicals in the environment make toxicology a very broad science. There are several fields of toxicology, including environmental (eg, air and water pollution), economic (eg, food additives, pesticides), legal (eg, forensics, regulation of emissions, and additives), laboratory (eg, analytical testing for chemicals), and biomedical (eg, toxicities of drugs used to treat disease in humans and animals).

The general principles of the toxic effects of chemicals are, for the most part, the same as the principles of the therapeutic effects of drugs.

GENERAL PRINCIPLES IN THE TREATMENT OF POISONING

Intentional and accidental poisonings are major medical problems. Every natural or synthetic chemical can cause injury if the dose is high enough.

The single most important treatment of poisoned patients is supportive care.

This is so important. You must treat the patient and not the poison. Provide airway support and ventilation and support blood pressure if needed. Toxicology screens of blood or urine take time and rarely change your therapy. If you know the poison, great; if not, treat the patient.

> To reduce absorption in an alert, relatively asymptomatic patient, use activated charcoal.

Three procedures are widely used to reduce the absorption of poisons from the GI tract: inducing emesis, gastric lavage, and activated charcoal. To be effective, emesis must be induced within 1 hour of ingestion, and it works best if induced within 5 minutes of ingestion. Gastric lavage needs to be carried out within 1 hour of ingestion. Emesis induced with ipecac and gastric lavage only empties the stomach. Any poison that has moved into the small intestine is not removed. Activated charcoal remains in the GI tract, absorbing poison throughout.

To enhance elimination, a number of techniques can be used. Multiple doses of charcoal reduce the half-life and increase clearance. Increasing the pH of the urine enhances elimination of weak acids. Hemodialysis and hemoperfusion can be used to help remove specific agents from the blood.

SPECIFIC ANTIDOTES

For some overdoses and poisons, specific antidotes are available. These are prime exam material and are relatively easy to learn (some you already know).

Toxin	Antidote
acetaminophen	N-acetylcysteine
arsenic, mercury, gold	BAL (dimercaprol)
β-blocker	glucagon
benzodiazepines	flumazenil
carbon monoxide	oxygen, hyperbaric oxygen
coumarin	vitamin K
cyanide	nitrites
digoxin	digoxin-specific Fab fragments
ethylene glycol or methanol	fomepizole
heparin	protamine
iron	deferoxamine
isoniazid	pyridoxine
lead	dimercaprol, penicillamine, or succimer
narcotics	naloxone
nitrites	methylene blue
organophosphates	atropine, pralidoxime

Scan through this list and pick out the ones you already know. You should remember that flumazenil is the benzodiazepine receptor antagonist and that naloxone is the narcotic antagonist. You should know from biochemistry that oxygen and carbon monoxide compete for the same site on hemoglobin. You should remember from autonomics that pralidoxime rescues the acetylcholinesterase enzyme from the organophosphates. You should already know that vitamin K is the antidote for coumarin overdose, and protamine is the antidote for heparin overdose. So, there are really only a few new ones here.

Some of the antidotes directly bind or neutralize the poison. For instance BAL (dimercaprol) chelates the metals, deferoxamine binds to iron, the monoclonal antibody to digoxin binds to the digoxin, and the nitrites neutralize cyanide. Dimercaprol, penicillamine, or succimer will all chelate lead. Both ethylene glycol and methanol are oxidized by alcohol dehydrogenase to toxic compounds. Fomepizole is a specific alcohol dehydrogenase inhibitor.

Index

abacavir, 163
abarelix, 179, 194
abatacept, 221
ABBOKINASE (urokinase), 83
abciximab, 80
ABILIFY (aripiprazole), 107
acarbose, 201–202
ACCUPRIL (quinapril), 63
ACE, 59–60, 62–64, 67, 70
acebutolol, 55, 67
ACEON (perindopril), 63
acetaminophen, 120, 220, 229
acetophenazine, 107
acetylcholine, 30–34, 36, 38–39, 41–43,
    45–46, 91, 108, 143, 213
acetylcholinesterase, 32, 38–39, 42, 230
ACHROMYCIN (tetracycline), 135,
    144–145
ACIPHEX (rabeprazole), 212
ACOVA (aripiprazole), 107
acrivastine, 205
ACTH, 186
actinomycin, 173, 176
ACTIVASE (alteplase), 83–84
active transport, 11, 175
ACTONEL (risedronate), 226
ACTOS (pioglitazone), 201
acyclovir, 165
adalimumab, 215
adefovir, 165
ARD (adenosine), 72, 78, 80, 163
adenosine, 72, 78, 80, 163
adrenal medulla, 32, 34, 47 186, 189
adrenaline, 32
ADRIAMYCIN (doxorubicin),
    173–174, 176
AFINITOR (everolimus), 180, 223–224
AGRYLIN (anagrelide), 80
agonist, 5–10, 40, 45, 48–52, 55, 66, 68,
    72, 91, 98–99, 101, 111, 117–121, 191,
    194, 201, 209, 226
AIDS, 163
akathisia, 107–108
AKINETON (biperiden), 112
ALDACTONE (spironolactone), 188

ALDOMET (methyldopa), 67
aldosterone, 62–64, 186, 188
alemtuzumab, 178
alendronate, 226
alfentanil, 117
alfuzosin, 53
ALINIA (nitazoxanide), 167
aliskiren, 64
alkylating agents, 171, 175, 178
ALLEGRA (fexofenadine), 206–207
allergy, penicillin, 139
allopurinol, 222
almotriptan, 222
alosetron, 215
ALOXI (palonosetron), 173
alprazolam, 98
ALTABAX (retapamulin), 135
ALTACE (ramipril), 63
alteplase, 83–84
aluminum, 213
ALVESCO (ciclesonide), 209
alvimopan, 117
ALUPENT (metaproterenol), 49
amantadine, 164
AMARYL (glimepiride), 201
ambenonium, 40–41
AMBIEN (zolpidem), 94, 98–99
ambrisentan, 211
AMERGE (naratriptan), 222
AMIDATE (etomidate), 123, 125
amikacin, 143, 151
AMIKIN (amikacin), 143, 151
amiloride, 60
aminoglutethimide, 188
aminoglycosides, 134–135, 142–146
aminosalicylic acid, 151
amiodarone, 77
amisulpride, 107
AMITIZA (lubiprostone), 214
amitriptyline, 101
amlodipine, 64
amobarbital, 94, 96
amoxicillin, 162
AMOXIL (amoxicillin), 138
amphetamine, 50

amphotericin B, 156–157
ampicillin, 138
ambrisentan, 211
AMYTAL (amobarbital), 94, 96
anabolic, 31–32, 190, 193
anagrelide, 80
anakinra, 221
anastrozole, 179
androgens, 189–190, 193
ANECTINE (succinylcholine), 46
ANGIOMAX (bivalirudin), 81,83
angiotensin, 59–60, 62
angiotensin converting enzyme, 62–63
anidulafungin, 156, 158
anistreplase, 83
antacids, 144, 213
ANTAGON (ganirelix), 194
antagonist, 5, 7–10, 42–43, 45–46, 52–54,
    56, 67, 80, 82, 91–92, 97, 101, 107–108,
    118, 120–121, 173, 179, 188, 190–191,
    194, 210–211, 213, 215, 221, 226, 229
anthracyclines, 171, 174, 176
anticoagulant, 69, 81–83
ANTILIRIUM (physostigmine), 40
antipsychotics, 52–53, 106–109
ANTISOL (fomepizole), 229–230
ANTIVERT (meclizine), 205–206
ANZEMET (dolasetron), 173
APIDRA (insulin glulisine), 200
aprepitant, 173
APTIVUS (tipranavir), 163
ara-A, 165
arachidonic acid, 80, 209, 217
ARALEN (chloroquine), 168–169
ARCOXIA (etoricoxib), 217
ardeparin, 81
ARDUAN (pipecuronium), 46
arecoline, 39
AREDIA (pamidronate), 226
arformoterol, 209
argatroban, 81
ARICEPT (donepezil), 40, 91
ARIMIDEX (anastrozole), 179
aripiprazole, 107
ARISTOCORT (triamcinolone), 186, 209

AROMASIN (exemestane), 179
articaine, 127
ARIXTRA (fondaparinux), 81, 83
arrhythmia, 78
arsenic, 229
ARSOBAL (melarsoprol), 167
artemether, 168
artemether-lumefantrine, 168
ARZERRA (ofatumumab), 178
asenapine, 107
ASMANEX TWISTHALER
   (mometasone), 209
asparaginase, 178
aspart, 200–201
aspirin, 69, 80, 120, 216–219
ASTELIN (azelastine), 205
astemizole, 206–207
asthma, 209–210
ATABRINE (quinacrine), 167
ATACAND (candesartan), 63
ATARAX (hydroxyzine), 205
atazanavir, 163
atenolol, 55, 67
ATIVAN (lorazepam), 94, 98
atomoxetine, 102
atovaquone, 167
atorvastatin, 86
atracurium, 46
atropine, 42–44, 78, 229
ATROVENT (ipratropium), 44–45, 210
aurothioglucose, 221
autonomic nervous system, 29
AVAPRO (irbesartan), 63
AVASTIN (bevacizumab), 178
AVINZA (morphine), 117–121
AVODART (dutasteride), 190, 194
AXERT (almotriptan), 222
AXID (nizatidine), 213
AZACTAM (aztreonam), 134, 136, 140
azathioprine, 214, 220, 223–224
azelastine, 205
AZILECT (rasagiline), 112
azithromycin, 145
AZLIN (azlocillin), 138
azlocillin, 138
AZMACORT (triamcinolone), 186, 209
azole antifungals, 155–156
aztreonam, 134, 136, 140
AZULFIDINE (sulfasalazine),
   148, 214, 220

bacitracin, 134, 136, 141
bactericidal, 132, 142, 150, 212
bacteriostatic, 132–133
BACTROBAN (mupirocin),135, 146
balsalazide, 214
BARACLUDE (entecavir), 165
barbiturates, 93–96, 125
barbiturates, withdrawal, 93–94, 96
basiliximab, 223–224
BAYCOL (cerivastatin), 86
BCNU (carmustine), 175
beclomethasone, 209

benazepril, 63
bendamustine, 175
BENICAR (olmesartan), 63
BENTYL (dicyclomine), 44
benzathine pen G, 138
benzocaine, 127
benzodiazepines, 93–94, 96–98
benztropine, 112
betamethasone, 186
BETAPACE (sotalol), 77
betaxolol, 55, 67
bethanechol, 39–40
bevacizumab, 178
BEXTRA (valdecoxib), 218
BEXXAR (tositumomab), 178
BIAXIN (clarithromycin), 143, 145
BILTRICIDE (praziquantel), 159–160
bioavailability, 11, 13–14, 82
biperiden, 112
bisacodyl, 214
bismuth, 212, 214
bismuth subsalicylate, 214
bisoprolol, 55, 67
bivalirudin, 81, 83
BLENOXANE (bleomycin), 174, 176–177
bleomycin, 174, 176–177
BONEFOS (clodronate), 226
BONINE (meclizine), 205–206
bortezomib, 171, 180–181
bosentan, 211
botulinum toxin, 46
BRETHAIRE (terbutaline), 49
BRETHINE (terbutaline), 49
bretylium, 77
BREVIBLOC (esmolol), 55, 67
BREVITAL (methohexital), 94, 96, 125
bromocriptine, 112
brompheniramine, 205
BROVANA (arformoterol), 209
budesonide, 209
bumetanide, 60
BUMEX (bumetanide), 60
bupivacaine, 127
buprenorphine, 117
bupropion, 101, 104
BUSPAR (buspirone), 101, 104
buspirone, 101, 104
BUTAZOLID (phenylbutazone), 216
butoconazole, 155
butorphanol, 117
BYETTA (exenatide), 201–202
BYSTOLIC (nebivolol), 67

CAFERGOT (ergotamine), 112, 222
CALAN (verapamil), 64
calcitonin, 225, 227
calcium channel blockers, 59–60, 64–65,
   69, 73, 77
calcium polycarbophil, 214
CAMPATH (alemtuzumab), 178
CAMPTOSAR (irinotecan), 176–177
CANCIDAS (caspofungin), 156, 158
candesartan, 63

CAPASTAT (capreomycin), 151
capecitabine, 176
CAPOTEN (captopril), 63
capreomycin, 151
captopril, 63
CARAFATE (sucralfate), 63
carbachol, 63
carbamazepine, 105, 114–115
carbenicillin, 138
carbidopa, 111–112
CARBOCAINE (mepivacaine), 127
carboplatin, 175
CARDENE (nicardipine), 64
cardiotoxicity, 174
CARDIZEM (diltiazem), 64
CARDURA (doxazosin), 53–54, 66
carmustine, 175
carteolol, 55
CARTROL (carteolol), 55
carvedilol, 56, 67
caspofungin, 156, 158
catabolic, 31
CATAPRES (clonidine), 48–49, 52,
   59–60, 67–68
catecholamine, 33, 49
CCNU (lomustine), 175
CECLOR (cefaclor), 139–140
CEFACLOR, 139–140
CEFAMANDOLE, 139
CEFAZOLIN, 139
cefepime, 139
CEFOTAXIME, 139
CEFOXITIN, 139
cefpirome, 139
CEFTRIAXONE, 139
CELEBREX (celecoxib), 218
celecoxib, 218
CELEXA (citalopram), 101
cell cycle, 171–172, 180–181
CELLCEPT (mycophenolate), 223
CENTAXARIN (ardeparin), 81
CEPHALEXIN, 139–140
cephalosporins, 134, 136–137,
   139–140
CEREBYX (fosphenytoin), 116
cerivastatin, 86
CESAMET (nabilone), 173
cestodes, 159–160
CERTICAN (everolimus), 180, 223–224
certolizumab pegol, 215
cetirizine, 206–207
cetrorelix, 194
CETROTIDE (cetrorelix), 194
cetuximab, 178
cevimeline, 39
charcoal, 229
CHEMET (succimer), 229–230
CHIROCAINE (levobupivacaine), 127
chlamydia, 144–145
chloral hydrate, 94
chlorambucil, 175
chloramphenicol, 135, 142, 146
chlordiazepoxide, 94, 97–98

CHLOROMYCETIN (chloramphenicol), 135, 142, 146
chloroquine, 168–169
chlorothiazide, 60
chlorpheniramine, 205
chlorprocaine, 127
chlorpromazine, 107–108
CHLORTRIMETON (chlorpheniramine), 205
chlotetracycline, 127
cholera, 144
cholesterol, 86–88, 157, 188
cholesterol synthesis, 87
cholestyramine, 87–88
cholinesterases, 38–39, 91
cholinomimetics, 38, 44
ciclesonide, 209
cidofovir, 165
cilastatin, 140
cilostazol, 84
cimetidine, 213
CIMZIA (certolizumab pegol), 215
cinchonism, 169
CIOVAN (valsartan), 63
CIPRO (ciprofloxacin), 149
ciprofloxacin, 149
cisapride, 213
cisatracurium, 46
cisplatin, 174
citalopram, 101
cladribine, 176
CLAFORAN (cefotaxime), 176
CLARINEX (desloratadine), 206–207
clarithromycin, 143
clearance, 14–15, 153, 229
clemastine, 206
CLEOCIN (clindamycin), 135, 142–143, 146
clevidipine, 64
CLEVIPREX (clevidipine), 64
clindamycin, 135, 142–143, 146
CLINORIL (sulindac), 216
clodronate, 226
CLOMID (clomiphene), 189, 191
clomiphene, 189, 191
clonazepam, 94, 116
clonidine, 48–49, 52, 59–60, 67–68
clopidogrel, 80
clorazepate, 94
clotrimazole, 155
cloxacillin, 138
clozapine, 107, 109
CLOZARIL (clozapine), 107, 109
COARTEM (artemether-lumefantrine), 168
cocaine, 127
codeine, 117, 119
COGENTIN (benztropine), 44, 112
COGNEX (tacrine), 40, 42, 91
COLASE (docusate), 214
COLAZAL (balsalazide), 214
colchicine, 221

colesevelam, 87, 201
COLESTID (colestipol), 87–88
colestipol, 87–88
COMPAZINE (prochlorperazine), 107
competitive antagonist, 8–9, 43, 92, 179, 194, 206, 211
COMT, 33, 48, 111
COMTAN (entacapone), 111
CORDARONE (amiodarone), 77
COREG (carvedilol), 56, 67
CORGARD (nadolol), 55, 67
CORLOPAM (fenoldopam), 66
cortisol, 186–187
CORVERT (ibutilide), 77
COSMEGEN (dactinomycin), 173, 176
COUMADIN (warfarin), 80–82
coumarin, 229–230
COZAAR (losartan), 63
craniosacral, 31–32
CRESTOR (rosuvastatin), 86
CRIXIVAN (indinavir), 163
Crohn's disease, 214–215
cross-dependence, 94
cross-tolerance, 93–94
CRYSTODIGIN (digitoxin), 71
CUBICIN (daptomycin), 134, 136, 141
CUTOXAN (cyclophosphamide), 173–175
cyanide, 66, 229–230
cyanocobalamin, 85
cyclooxygenase, 80, 217, 219
cyclopentolate, 44
cyclophosphamide, 173–175
cycloserine, 151
cyclosporine, 214, 220
CYMBALTA (duloxetine), 101–102
cyproheptadine, 206
cyproterone, 190, 194
CYTADREN (aminoglutethimide), 188
cytarabine, 176
CYTOSAR-U (cytarabine), 176
CYTOTEC (misoprostol), 192, 213, 218
CYTOVENE (ganciclovir), 165

dabigatran, 81
daclizumab, 223–224
dactinomycin, 173, 176
dalfopristin, 145
DALGAN (dezocine), 117
dalteparin, 81
danthron, 214
dantrolene, 46
dapsone, 151, 153–154
DARAPRIM (pyrimethamine), 147, 168
darifenacin, 44
darunavir, 163
DARVON (propoxyphene), 118
dasatinib, 180
daunomycin, 176
daunorubicin, 174, 176
DAYPRO (oxaprozin), 216
DECADRON (dexamethasone), 186

DECLOMYCIN (demeclocycline), 144
deferoxamine, 229–230
degarelix, 179, 194
dehydroemetine, 167
delavirdine, 163
DEMADEX (torsemide), 60
demecarium, 40
demeclocycline, 144
DEMEROL (meperidine), 118–120
denosumab, 227
DEPAKOTE (valproate), 105, 114
dependence, 36, 93–94, 97–98
DEPO-MEDROL (methylprednisolone), 186
deprenyl, 112
desipramine, 101–102
desirudin, 81, 83
deslansoprazole, 212
desloratadine, 206
desvenlafaxine, 101–102
DESYREL (trazodone), 101, 104
DETROL (tolterodine), 44
dexamethasone, 186
dexmethylphenidate, 50
DEXEDRINE (amphetamine), 50
dexrazoxane, 177
diabetes insipidus, 105, 199
diabetes mellitus, 199
diabetics, 54
diazepam, 64, 94, 97–98
DIBENZYLINE (phenoxybenzamine), 53
diclofenac, 216
dicloxacillin, 138
dicumarol, 81
dicyclomine, 44
didanosine, 163
DIDRONAL (etidronate), 226
diethylcarbamazine, 159–161
diethylstilbestrol, 189, 191
DIFLUCAN (fluconazole), 155–156
digitalis, 71
digitoxin, 71
digoxin, 71, 78, 229–230
dihydrocodeine, 117
dihydroergotamine, 222
DILANTIN (phenytoin), 74, 115–116
DILAUDID (hydromorphone), 118
diltiazem, 64
dimenhydrinate, 205–206
dimercaprol, 229–230
DIMETABS (dimenhydrinate), 205–206
DIPENTUM (olsalazine), 214
diphenhydramine, 205–206
diphenoxylate, 120, 214
diphtheria, 145
DIPRIVAN (propofol), 123, 125
dipyridamole, 80
dirithromycin, 145
disopyramide, 74–75
DISTOCIDE (praziquantel), 159–160
DITROPAN (oxybutynin), 44
diuretics, 59–62, 66, 70–71
DIURIL (chlorothiazide), 60

dobutamine, 49, 72
DOBUTREX (dobutamine), 49, 72
docetaxel, 176–177
dofetilide, 77
dolasetron, 173
DOLOPHINE (methadone), 118, 120
DOMALIN (quazepam), 94
donepezil, 40, 91
dopamine, 33, 47, 49–50, 66, 72, 91, 98, 101, 103–104, 106–112, 213
DORIBAX (doripenem), 140
doripenem, 140
doxacurium, 46
doxazosin, 53–54, 66
doxercalciferol, 198
doxorubicin, 173–174, 176
doxycycline, 144, 168
DRAMAMINE (dimenhydrinate), 205–206
dronedarone, 77
drotrecogin alfa, 81, 83
DTIC-DOME (dacarbazine), 175
DULCOLAX (bisacodyl), 214
duloxetine, 101–102
DURANEST (etidocaine), 127
dutasteride, 190, 194
DYNABAC (dirithromycin), 145
DYNACIRC (isradipine), 64
dystonia, 107

echothiophate, 40
econazole, 155
EDECRIN (ethacrynic acid), 60
edrophonium, 40–41
efavirenz, 163
efficacy, 6
EFFIENT (prasugrel), 80
ELAVIL (amitriptyline), 101
ELDEPRYL (selegiline or deprenyl), 112
eletriptan, 222
ELIDEL (pimecrolimus), 223
ELLENC (epirubicin), 176
ELOXATIN (oxaliplatin), 175
ELSPAR (asparaginase), 178
EMEND (aprepitant), 173
emetine, 167
EMINASE (anistreplase), 83
emtricitabine, 163
EMTRIVA (emtricitabine), 163
ENABLEX (darifenacin), 44
enalapril, 63
ENBREL (etanercept), 221
endometriosis, 192, 194
enflurane, 122–123
enfuvirtide, 163–164
enoxacin, 149
enoxaparin, 81
entacapone, 111
entecavir, 165
ENTEREG (alvimopan), 117, 119
ephedrine, 50
epilepsy, 94, 96, 113, 115
epinephrine, 8, 32–33, 47–51, 78, 186, 209

epirubicin, 176
EPIVIR (lamivudine), 163, 165
eplerenone, 60, 64
epoprostenol, 211
eprosartan, 63
EQUETRO (carbamazepine), 105, 114–115
ERAXIS (anidulafungin), 156, 158
ERBITUX (cetuximab), 178
ERCAF (ergotamine), 112, 222
ERGOMAR (ergotamine), 112, 222
ergosterol, 156–158
ergotamine, 112, 222
erlotinib, 180
ertapenem, 140
ERYCETTE (erythromycin), 135, 142–143, 145–146
erythromycin, 135, 142–143, 145–146
erythropoietin, 85, 173
escitalopram, 101
esmolol, 55, 67
esomeprazole, 212
estradiol, 189–191
estriol, 189, 191
estrogen, 24, 179–180, 191–194
estrone, 189, 191
eszopiclone, 94, 98
etanercept, 221
ethacrynic acid, 60
ethambutol, 151, 153
ethanol, 94
ethinyl estradiol, 189
ethionamide, 151
ethosuximide, 114–115
ethmozine (moricizine), 75
ETHRANE (enflurane), 122–123
ethylene glycol, 229–230
etidocaine, 127
etidronate, 226
etodolac, 216
etomidate, 123, 125
etoposide, 176–177
etoricoxib, 218
etravirine, 163
EULEXIN (flutamide), 190
EUTHROID (liotrix), 197
everolimus, 180, 223–224
EVISTA (raloxifene), 189, 191, 226
EVOXAC (cevimeline), 39
EXANTA (ximelagatran), 84
EXELON (rivastigmine), 40, 91
exemestane, 179
exenatide, 201–202
EXLAX (phenolphthalein), 214
extrapyramidal effects, 108
ezetimibe, 87–88

FANAPT (iloperidone), 107
famciclovir, 165
famotidine, 213
FAMVIR (famciclovir), 165
FARESTON (toremifene), 179, 189, 191
FASLODEX (fulvestrant), 179
febuxostat, 221

felbamate, 115
FELBATOL (felbamate), 115
FELDENE (piroxicam), 216
felodipine, 64
FEMSTAT (butoconazole), 155
fenoldopam, 66
fenoprofen, 217
fentanyl, 117, 120
fesoterodine, 44
fexofenadine, 206–207
filaria, 159–160
filgrastim, 173
finasteride, 190, 194
FIRMAGON (degarelix), 179, 194
FLAGYL (metronidazole), 166–167
flecainide, 75
FLOLAN (epoprostenol), 211
FLOMAX (tamsulosin), 53–54
fluconazole, 155–156
FLUMADINE (rimantadine), 164
flumazenil, 97
FLUOTHANE (halothane), 122–123
fluoxymesterone, 190
fluphenazine, 108
flutamide, 190
FOCALIN (dexmethylphenidate), 50
folate antagonists, 135, 147
folic acid, 85, 134, 147, 154, 175
fomepizole, 229
fondaparinux, 81, 83
FORADIL (formoterol), 209
FORANE (isoflurane), 122
formaldehyde, 150
formestane, 179
formoterol, 209
FORTEO (teriparatide), 198, 227
FORTOVASE (saquinavir), 163
FOSAMAX (alendronate), 226
fosamprenavir, 163
fosfomycin, 134
fosinopril, 63
fosphenytoin, 116
FRAGMIN (dalteparin), 81
FROVA (frovatriptan), 222
frovatriptan, 222
fulvestrant, 179
FULVIN (griseofulvin), 156
FUNGIZONE (amphotericin), 157
furosemide, 60
FUZEON (enfuvirtide), 163

GABA, 9, 95–96, 98
gabapentin, 115
GABITRIL (tiagabine), 116
galantamine, 40, 91
gallamine, 46
ganciclovir, 165
ganirelix, 194
GANTANEL (sulfamethoxazole), 134, 148
GARAMYCIN (gentamicin), 143
gastric lavage, 229
gemcitabine, 176
gemtuzumab ozogamicin, 178

GEMZAR (gemcitabine), 176
gentamicin, 143
GEOPEN (carbenicillin), 138
glargine, 200
glaucoma, 41
GLEEVEC (imatinib), 171
glimepiride, 201
glipizide, 201
glomerular filtration, 25
glucagon, 199
glucocorticoids, 179
GLUCOPHAGE (metformin), 201
GLUCOTROL (glipizide), 201
glyburide, 201
glycopyrrolate, 44
glycosides, cardiac, 69
GLYSET (miglitol), 201
gold, 220
gold sodium thiomalate, 221
golimumab, 221
goserelin, 194
GOTAMINE (ergotamine), 222
granisetron, 173
GRIFULVIN (griseofulvin), 156
griseofulvin, 158
growth factors, 173
guanabenz, 52, 68
guanfacine, 52

HALCION (triazolam), 94
HALDOL (haloperidol), 107
half-life, 111
haloperidol, 107
HALOTESTIN (fluoxymesterone), 190
halothane, 122
headaches, 216
HECTOROL (doxercalciferol), 198
helminths, 159
heparin, 81–82, 229–230
HEPSERA (adefovir), 165
HERCEPTIN (trastuzumab), 178
heroin, 117, 119–120
hirudin, 81
HISMANAL (astemizole), 206
histamine, 205
HIV, 162
HMG CoA reductase, 86
hookworm, 160
HUMIRA (adalimumab), 215, 221
HUMORSOL (demecarium), 40
HUMULIN (insulin), 199
hydralazine, 66, 70
HYDREA (hydroxyurea), 178
hydrochlorothiazide, 60
hydrocodone, 118
hydrocortisone, 186
hydromorphone, 118
hydroxychloroquine, 168
hydroxyprogesterone, 190
hydroxyurea, 178
hydroxyzine, 205
hypercalcemia, 177
HYTRIN (terazosin), 53–54, 66

ibritumomab tiuxetan, 178
ibuprofen, 216
ibutilide, 77
IDAMYCIN (idarubicin), 176
idarubicin, 176
IFEX (ifosfamide), 175
ifosfamide, 175
iloperidone, 107
iloprost, 211
ILOTYCIN (erythromycin), 135
imatinib, 171
imipenem, 136, 140
imipramine, 101
IMITREX (sumatriptan), 222
IMODIUM (loperamide), 120
IMURAN (azathioprine), 214, 220
inamrinone, 72
indapamide, 60
INDERAL (propranolol), 55, 67, 76
indinavir, 163
INDOCIN (indomethacin), 216
indomethacin, 216
influenza, 164
infusion rate, 66
INH (isoniazid), 133
inhibitory concentration, 134
INNOHEP (tinzaparin), 81
INOCOR (inamrinone), 72
INSPRA (eplerenone), 60, 64
insulin, 199
insulin detemir, 200
insulin glulisine, 200
INTELENCE (etravirine), 163
INVEGA (paliperidone), 107
inverse agonist, 9
INVANZ (ertapenem), 140
INVIRASE (saquinavir), 163
iodoquinol, 167
ipecac, 229
ipratropium, 44–45, 210
irbesartan, 63
irinotecan, 176
iron, 85, 177, 229–230
ISENTRESS (raltegravir), 163
isocarboxazid, 101, 103
isoflurane, 122
isoniazid, 133, 152
isoproterenol, 47, 49–52, 78
ISOPTIN (verapamil), 64
isosorbide dinitrate, 65
isosorbide mononitrate, 65
isradipine, 64
ISTODAX (romidepsin), 181
ISUPREL (isoproterenol), 47
itraconazole, 155
ivermectin, 159–161
ixabepilone, 177
IXEMPRA (ixabepilone), 177

JANUVIA (sitagliptin), 201–202

KABIKINASE (streptokinase), 83
KALETRA (lopinavir), 163

kanamycin, 143, 151
KANTREX (kanamycin), 143, 151
KAPIDEX (deslansoprazole), 212
KEFLEX (cephalexin), 139
KEPPRA (levetiracetam), 114
KERLONE (betaxolol), 55
KETALAR (ketamine), 123
ketamine, 123
KETEK (telithromycin), 145
ketoconazole, 155, 188
ketolide, 135
ketoprofen, 217
ketorolac, 216, 218
KINERET (anakinra), 221
KLONOPIN (clonazepam), 94, 116
KYTRIL (granisetron), 173

labetalol, 55–56, 67
lacosamide, 116
LAMICTAL (lamotrigine), 105, 114
LAMISIL (terbinafine), 158
lamivudine, 163, 165
lamotrigine, 105, 114
LAMPIT (nifurtimox), 167
lanoteplase, 83
LANOXIN (digoxin), 71, 229–230
lansoprazole, 212
lapatinib, 178
LASIX (furosemide), 60
LENTARIN (formestane), 179
LENTE (insulin), 199
lepirudin, 81
leprosy, 151
LETAIRIS (ambrisentan), 211
leucovorin, 175
LEUKERAN (chlorambucil), 175
leuprolide, 179, 194
LEUSTATIN (cladribine), 176
LEVATOL (penbutolol), 55, 67
LEVEMIR (insulin glulisine), 200
levetiracetam, 114
LEVO-DROMORAN (levorphanol), 118
levobunolol, 55
levobupivacaine, 127
levocetirizine, 206
levodopa, 111
levonorgestrol, 190
LEVOPHED (norepinephrine), 8, 32–33,
    35, 37, 47
levorphanol, 118
LEVOTHYROID (thyroxine), 197
levothyroxine, 197
LEVOXINE (thyroxine), 197
LEXAPRO (escitalopram), 101
LEXIVA (fosamprenavir), 163
LIBRIUM (chlordiazepoxide), 94
lidocaine, 74, 127
lincomycin, 146
linezolid, 145
liothyronine, 197
liotrix, 197
LIPITOR (atorvastatin), 86
lipoprotein, 86

liraglutide, 201
lisinopril, 63
lispro, 200
lithium, 105
LODINE (etodolac), 216
log kill, 172
LOMOTIL (diphenoxylate), 214
lomustine, 175
loop diuretics, 60
LOPAMAX (topiramate), 116
loperamide, 120
lopinavir, 163
LOPRESSOR (metoprolol), 55
LORABID (loracarbef), 140
loracarbef, 140
loratadine, 206
lorazepam, 94, 98
losartan, 63
LOTENSIN (benazepril), 63
LOTRIMIN (clotrimazole), 155
LOTRONEX (alosetron), 215
lovastatin, 86
LOVENOX (enoxaparin), 81
loxapine, 107
LOZOL (indapamide), 60
lubiprostone, 214
LUDIOMIL (maprotiline), 101
LUNESTA (eszopiclone), 94
LUPRON (leuprolide), 179, 194
Lyme disease, 144
LYSODREN (mitotane), 178

MAC, 124
macrolides, 135, 145
major tranquilizers, 106
malaria, 167
malathion, 40
MANDOL (cefamandole), 139
MAO, 145
MAO inhibitors, 103–104
maprotiline, 101
maraviroc, 163
MARCAINE (bupivacaine), 127
MAREZINE (cyclizine), 206
MARPLAN (isocarboxazid), 101
MATULANE (procarbazine), 178
MAXAIRE (pirbuterol), 209
MAZALT (rizatriptan), 222
mebendazole, 159
mechlorethamine, 175
meclizine, 205
meclofenamate, 216
medroxyprogesterone, 190
MEFOXIN (cefoxitin), 139
megestrol, 190
melagatran, 84
melarsoprol, 167
MELLARIL (thioridazine), 107
meloxicam, 217
melphalan, 175
memantine, 91
meperidine, 118
MEPHYTON (vitamin K), 140, 229

mepivacaine, 127
MEPRON (atovaquone), 167
mercaptopurine, 176
mercury, 229
MERIDIA (sibutramine), 104
meropenem, 140
MERREM (meropenem), 140
mesalamine, 214
mesoridazine, 107
MESTINON (pyridostigmine), 40
mestranol, 189
metabolism, 11, 24, 196
METAMUCIL (psyllium), 214
METAPREL (metaproterenol), 49
metaproterenol, 49
metformin, 201
methacholine, 39
methadone, 118, 120
methanol, 229
methenamine, 150
methicillin, 138
methimazole, 197
methohexital, 94, 96
methotrexate, 147, 173–175, 214, 220
methoxyflurane, 122
methylcellulose, 214
methyldopa, 67
methylnaltrexone, 118
methylphenidate, 50
methylprednisolone, 186
methyltestosterone, 190
metoclopramide, 213
metocurine iodide, 46
metolazone, 60
metoprolol, 55
metronidazole, 166
metyrapone, 188
MEVACOR (lovastatin), 86
MEXATE (methotrexate), 147, 173–175, 214, 220
mexiletine, 74
MEXITIL (mexiletine), 74
MIACALCIN (calcitonin), 227
MIC, 134
MICARDIS (telmisartan), 63
miconazole, 155
MICRONASE (glyburide), 201
microtubules, 177
midazolam, 125
mifepristone, 190, 192
miglitol, 201
migraines, 216
MIGRANAL (dihydroergotamine), 222
milnacipran, 101
milrinone, 72
mineralocorticoids, 188
MINIPRESS (prazosin), 53–54, 66
MINOCIN (minocycline), 144
minocycline, 144
minoxidil, 66
miosis, 36
MIRAPEX (pramipexole), 112
mirtazapine, 101, 104

misoprostol, 192, 213, 218
MITHRACIN (plicamycin), 176
mithramycin, 176–177
mitomycin, 176
mitotane, 178
mitoxantrone, 178
MIVACRON (mivacurium), 46
mivacurium, 46
MOBIC (meloxicam), 217
MODANE (danthron), 214
moexipril, 63
mometasone, 209
MONISTAT (miconazole), 155
monobactam, 140
MONOPRIL (fosinopril), 63
montelukast, 209
MONUROL (fosfomycin), 134
moricizine, 75
morphine, 118
motion sickness, 206
MOTRIN (ibuprofen), 216
MOXOBIL (plerixafor), 173
MULTAQ (dronedarone), 77
mupirocin, 135
muromonab, 223
muscarine, 39
muscarinic, 39–43
MUSTARGEN (mechlorethamine), 175
MUTAMYCIN (mitomycin), 176
MYAMBUTOL (ethambutol), 153
myasthenia gravis, 40, 223
MYCELEX (clotrimazole), 155
mycobacteria, 151
MYCOBUTIN (rifabutin), 151
mycophenolate mofetil, 224
mycoplasma, 144
MYCOSTATIN (nystatin), 156–157
mydriasis, 36
MYLOTARG (gemtuzumab ozogamicin), 178

N-acetylcysteine, 220
nabilone, 173
nabumetone, 216
nadolol, 55, 67
nafarelin, 194
NAFCIL (nafcillin), 138
nafcillin, 138
nalbuphine, 117
NALFON (fenoprofen), 217
nalidixic acid, 150
nalmefene, 117
naloxone, 7, 117–118, 229
naltrexone, 118
NAMENDA (memantine), 91
NAPROSYN (naproxen), 216
naproxen, 216
naratriptan, 222
NARCAN (naloxone), 229
narcotic, withdrawal, 119
narcotics, 117
NARDIL (phenelzine), 101
natalizumab, 215

nateglinide, 201
NATRECOR (nesiritide), 70
NAVANE (thiothixene), 107
NAVELBINE (vinorelbine), 176
NEBCIN (tobramycin), 143
nebivolol, 67
nefazodone, 101, 104
nematodes, 160
NEMBUTAL (pentobarbital), 94
neomycin, 143
NEOSPORIN (bacitracin), 134
neostigmine, 40
NEOSYNEPHRINE (phenylephrine), 48
nephrotoxicity, 62
nesiritide, 70
netilmicin, 143
NETROMYCIN (netilmicin), 143
NEUPOGEN (filgrastim), 173
NEUPRO (rotigotine), 112
neuraminidase, 164
neuroleptic malignant syndrome, 109
neuroleptics, 106
NEURONTIN (gabapentin), 115–116
neurotoxicity, 143, 174
nevirapine, 163
NEXAVAR (sorafenib), 180
NEXIUM (esomeprazole), 212
niacin, 87
nicardipine, 64
nicotine, 40
nicotinic, 40
nifedipine, 64
nifurtimox, 167
NILANDRON (nilutamide), 179, 190
nilotinib, 180
nilutamide, 179, 190
NIMBEX (cisatracurium), 46
nisoldipine, 64
nitazoxanide, 167
nitrates, 65, 195
nitrogen mustards, 171
nitroglycerin, 65
nitroprusside, 66, 70
nitrous oxide, 122–124
nizatidine, 213
NIZORAL (ketoconazole), 155
NOLVADEX (tamoxifen), 179
noncompetitive antagonist, 8
noradrenaline, 32
NORCURON (vecuronium), 46
norepinephrine, 33, 35, 50
norethindrone, 190
NORMODYNE (labetalol), 55
NORPACE (disopyramide), 74
NORPLANT (levonorgestrol), 190
NORPRAMIN (desipramine), 101
nortriptyline, 101
NORVASC (amlodipine), 64
NORVIR (ritonavir), 163
NOVANTRONE (mitoxantrone), 178
NOVOCAINE (procaine), 127
NOXAFIL (posaconazole), 155
NPH (insulin), 199

NSAID, 213, 217
NUBAIN (nalbuphine), 117
NUCYNTA (tapentadol), 117
NUPRINM (ibuprofen), 216
NUROMAX (doxacurium), 46
nystatin, 156

octreotide, 213
ofatumumab, 178
olanzapine, 107
olmesartan, 63
olopatadine, 206
olsalazine, 214
omalizumab, 210
omeprazole, 212
OMNARIS (ciclesonide), 209
OMNIPEN (ampicillin), 138
ONCOVIN (vincristine), 173
ondansetron, 173
OPANA (oxymorphone), 118
opiates, 117
optic neuritis, 153
oral contraceptives, 192
ORENCIA (abatacept), 221
orlistat, 215
ORTHOCLONE OKT3 (muromonab), 223
ORUDIS (ketoprofen), 217
oseltamivir, 164
osteoporosis, 188
ototoxicity, 62, 141, 143
oxacillin, 138
oxaliplatin, 175
oxaprozin, 216
oxazepam, 94
oxazolidinone, 135
oxcarbazepine, 114
oxiconazole, 155
OXISTAT (oxiconzaole), 186
oxybutynin, 44
oxycodone, 118
OXYCONTIN (oxycodone), 118
oxymorphone, 118
oxytetracycline, 144

PABA, 147
paclitaxel, 176–177
paliperidone, 107
palivizumab, 165
palonosetron, 173
pamidronate, 226
pancuronium, 46
panitumumab, 178
pantoprazole, 212
PARAPLATIN (carboplatin), 175
parasympathetic, 31, 210
parathion, 40
paricalcitol, 198
parkinsonism, 107
PARLODEL (bromocriptine), 112
PARNATE (tranylcypromine), 100
paroxetine, 101
partial agonist, 6
partial pressure, 123

passive diffusion, 25
PATANASE (olopatadine), 206
PATHOCIL (dicloxacillin), 138
PAVULON (pancuronium), 46
PAXIL (paroxetine), 101
pazopanib, 180
peginterferon, 165
penbutolol, 55, 67
PENETREX (enoxacin), 149
penicillamine, 229
penicillin G, 138
penicillin V, 138
penicillin-binding proteins, 136
penicillins, 138
PENTAM (pentamidine), 167
pentazocine, 117–118, 121
PENTIDS (penicillin G), 138
pentobarbital, 94
PENTOSTAM (sodium stibogluconate), 167
pentostatin, 176
PENTOTHAL (thiopental), 94
pentoxifylline, 84
PEPCID (famotidine), 213
PEPTO-BISMOL, 212, 214
peramivir, 164
pergolide, 112
perindopril, 63
PERMAX (pergolide), 112
perphenazine, 107
pertussis, 145
phenelzine, 101, 103
phenobarbital, 94, 96
phenolphthalein, 214
phenoxybenzamine, 53
phentolamine, 53
phenylbutazone, 216
phenylephrine, 48
phenylpropanolamine, 50
phenytoin, 74, 115
phenytoin, kinetics, 115
PHOSPHOLINE (echothiophate), 40
photosensitivity, 144
physostigmine, 40
pilocarpine, 39
pimecrolimus, 223
pindolol, 55, 67
pinworm, 160
pioglitazone, 201
pipecuronium, 46
piperacillin, 138
PIPRACEL (piperacillin), 138
pirbuterol, 209
pirenzepine, 44
piroxicam, 216
PLAQUENIL (hydroxychloroquine), 168
plasmids, 133
plasmodium, 167
PLATINOL (cisplatin), 174
PLENAXIS (abarelix), 179, 194
PLENDIL (felodipine), 64
plerixafor, 173
PLETAL (cilostazol), 84

plicamycin, 176–177
poisoning, 228
polyene antifungals, 157
POLYSPORIN (bacitracin), 134
PONSTEL (mefenamic acid), 217
PONTOCAINE (tetracaine), 127
posaconazole, 155
postganglionic, 31
potency, 6
PRADAXA (dabigatran), 81
pralidoxime, 42, 229–230
pramipexole, 112
pramlintide, 201
PRANDIN (repaglinide), 201
prasugrel, 80
PRAVACHOL (pravastatin), 86
pravastatin, 86
prazosin, 53–54, 66
PRECOSE (acarbose), 201
prednisolone, 186
prednisone, 186
preganglionic, 31
PREVACID (lansoprazole), 212
PREZISTA (darunavir), 163
PRIFTIN (rifapentine), 151
prilocaine, 127
PRILOSEC (omeprazole), 212
PRIMACOR (milrinone), 72
primaquine, 168
PRINIVIL (lisinopril), 63
PRISCOLINE (tolazoline), 53
PRISTIQ (desvenlafaxine), 101
probenecid, 138, 222
procainamide, 74
procaine, 127
PROCAN (procainamide), 74
procarbazine, 178
PROCARDIA (nifedipine), 64
prochlorperazine, 107
progesterone, 190
PROGRAF (tacrolimus), 223
prolactin, 107
PROLIA (denosumab), 227
PROLIXIN (fluphenazine), 108
promethazine, 206
propafenone, 74
propantheline, 44
propofol, 123, 125
propoxyphene, 118
propranolol, 55, 67, 76
PROPULSID (cisapride), 213
propylthiouracil, 197
PROSCAR (finasteride), 190, 194
prostaglandin, 213
PROSTAPHLIN (oxacillin), 138
prostatic hypertrophy, 194
PROSTIGMIN (neostigmine), 40
protamine, 82, 200
protease inhibitors, 163
PROTONIX (pantoprazole), 212
PROTOPAM (pralidoxime), 229
PROTOSTAT (metronidazole), 166
PROVENTIL (albuterol), 49, 209

PROVOCHOLINE (methacholine), 39
psyllium, 214
PULMICORT (budesonide), 209
PURINETHOL (mercaptopurine), 214
pyrazinamide, 153
pyridostigmine, 40
pyridoxine, 152
pyrimethamine, 147, 168

quazepam, 94
QUELICIN (succinylcholine), 46
QUESTRAN (cholestyramine), 87
quetiapine, 107
quinacrine, 167
quinapril, 63
quinestrol, 189
quinidine, 74
quinine, 75, 168
quinolones, 149–150
quinupristin, 145
QVAR (beclomethasone), 209

radioactive iodine, 197
rabeprazole, 212
raloxifene, 189, 191, 226
raltegravir, 163
ramelteon, 94
ramipril, 63
RANEXA (ranolazine), 72
ranitidine, 213
ranolazine, 72
RAPAFLO (silodosin), 53
RAPAMUNE (sirolimus), 223
rasagiline, 112
reboxetine, 101
REFLUDAN (lepirudin), 81
REGITINE (phentolamine), 53
REGLAN (metoclopramide), 213
RELAFEN (nabumetone), 216
RELENZA (zanamivir), 164
RELISTOR (methylnaltrexone), 118
RELPAX (eletriptan), 222
REMERON (mirtazapine), 101
REMINYL (galantamine), 40
REMODULIN (treprostinil), 211
renin, 36
REOPRO (abciximab), 80
repaglinide, 201
REQUIP (ropinirole), 112
RESCRIPTOR (delavirdine), 163
resistance, bacterial, 132
respiratory syncytial virus, 165
RESTORIL (temazepam), 94
retapamulin, 135
reteplase, 83
RETROVIR (zidovudine), 163
retrovirus, 163
reverse transcriptase inhibitors, 163
REVEX (nalmefene), 117
REYATAZ (atazanavir), 163
ribavirin, 165
ribosomes, 142
ridogrel, 80

rifabutin, 151
RIFADIN (rifampin), 152
rifampin, 152
rifapentine, 151
RIFATER (pyrazinamide), 153
RIMACTANE (rifampin), 153
rimantadine, 164
risedronate, 226
RISPERDAL (risperidone), 107
risperidone, 109
RITALINE (methylphenidate), 50
ritonavir, 163
RITUXAN (rituximab), 178
rituximab, 178
rivastigmine, 40
rizatriptan, 222
ROBINUL (glycopyrrolate), 44
ROCEPHIN (ceftriaxone), 139
Rocky Mountain Spotted Fever, 144
rocuronium, 46
rofecoxib, 218
ROGAINE (minoxidil), 66
ROMAZICON (flumazenil), 97
romidepsin, 181
ropinirole, 112
ropivacaine, 127
rosiglitazone, 201
rosuvastatin, 86
rotigotine, 112
roundworms, 159
ROXANOL (morphine), 118
ROZEREM (ramelteon), 94
RUFEN (ibuprofen), 216
RYTHMOL (propafenone), 74

SALAGEN (pilocarpine), 39
salicylism, 219
salivary glands, 35
salmeterol, 209
SANDOSTATIN (octreotide), 213
SANCTURA (trospium), 44
SANDIMMUNE (cyclosporine), 214, 220
SAPHRIS (asenapine), 107
saquinavir, 163
sargramostim, 173
sarin, 40
SAVELLA (milnacipran), 101
schistosomiasis, 159
scopolamine, 44
secobarbital, 94
SECONAL (secobarbital), 94
SECTRAL (acebutolol), 55, 67
seizures, 96, 104, 113
selegiline, 112
SELZENTRY (maraviroc), 163
SEMILENTE (insulin), 199
SEMPREX-D (acrivastine), 205
senna, 214
SENSORCAINE (bupivacaine), 127
SERAX (oxazepam), 94
SEREVENT (salmeterol), 209
SERLECT (sertindole), 107
SEROMYCIN (cycloserine), 151

SEROQUEL (quetiapine), 107
SEPTOCAINE (articaine), 127
sertindole, 107
sertraline, 101
SERZONE (nefazodone), 101
sibutramine, 104
silodosin, 53
SIMULECT (basiliximab), 223
simvastatin, 86
SINEMET (carbidopa and levodopa), 111
SINEQUAN (doxepin), 101
SINGULAIR (montelukast), 209
sirolimus, 223
sitagliptin, 201
SKELID (tiludronate), 226
SLO-PHYLLIN (theophylline), 210
SOLGANGAL (aurothioglucose), 221
SOLIAN (amisulpride), 107
solifenacin, 44
soman, 40
SONATA (zaleplon), 94
sorafenib, 180
sotalol, 77
spectrum, 132
SPEXTAZOLE (econazole), 155
SPIRIVA (tiotropium), 45, 210
spirochetes, 144
spironolactone, 60, 188
SPORANOX (itraconazole), 155
SPRYCEL (dasatinib), 180
SSRIs, 101
STADOL (butorphanol), 117
STAPHCILLIN (methicillin), 138
STARLIX (nateglinide), 201
stavudine, 163
sterol, 157
stibogluconate, 167
STILPHOSTROL (diethylstilbestrol), 189
STRATTERA (atomoxetine), 102
streptogramin, 135
streptokinase, 83–84
streptomycin, 143, 151
SUBLIMAZE (fentanyl), 117
succimer, 229
succinylcholine, 46
sucralfate, 213
sufentanil, 118
sulbactam, 137
sulfacetamide, 148
sulfadiazine, 148
sulfamethoxazole, 148
sulfapyridine, 148
sulfasalazine, 148, 214
sulfonamides, 133
sulindac, 216
sumatriptan, 222
sunitinib, 180
superinfection, 133
suprofen, 217
suramin, 167
SUSTIVA (efavirenz), 163
SUTEN (sunitinib), 180
SYMLIN (pramlintide), 201

SYMMETREL (amantadine), 112
sympathetic, 31
SYNAGIS (palivizumab), 165
SYNAREL (nafarelin), 194
SYNERCID (dalfopristin, quinupristin), 145
SYNTHROID (thyroxine), 197

t-PA, 83–84
tacrine, 40
tacrolimus, 223
TAGAMET (cimetidine), 213
TALWIN (pentazocine), 117
TAMBOCOR (flecainide), 75
TAMIFLU (oseltamivir), 164
tamoxifen, 179, 189, 191
tamsulosin, 53
TAO (troleandomycin), 145
TAPAZOLE (methimazole), 197
tapentadol, 117
tapeworms, 159
TARCEVA (erlotinib), 180
tardive dyskinesia, 107
TASIGNA (nilotinib), 180
TAVIST (clemastine), 206
TAXOL (paclitaxel), 176
tazobactam, 137
TEGOPEN (cloxacillin), 138
TEGRETOL (carbamazepine), 105, 114
teicoplanin, 141
TEKTURNA (aliskiren), 64
telavancin, 141
telbivudine, 165
telithromycin, 145
telmisartan, 63
temazepam, 94
TEMODAR (temozolomide), 175
temozolomide, 175
TEMPRA (acetaminophen), 220
temsirolimus, 180
tenecteplase, 83
TENEX (guanfacine), 52, 68
teniposide, 176–177
tenofovir, 163
TENORMIN (atenolol), 55, 67
TENSILON (edrophonium), 40
TERAZOL (terconazole), 155
terazosin, 53–54, 66
terbinafine, 158
terbutaline, 49
terconazole, 155
teriparatide, 198, 227
TERRAMYCIN (oxytetracycline), 144
testolactone, 190
testosterone, 179, 190, 193–194
tetracaine, 127
tetracycline, 144–145
TEVETEN (eprosartan), 63
thalidomide, 154
THEO-DUR (theophylline), 210
therapeutic index, 7
therapeutic window, 7
thiazide diuretics, 60

THIOGUAN (thioguanine), 176
thioguanine, 176
thiopental, 94, 96, 123
thioridazine, 107
thiotepa, 175
thiothixene, 107
thoracolumbar, 31
THORAZINE (chlorpromazine), 107
thyroglobulin, 196
THYROLAR (liotrix), 197
tiagabine, 116
TICAR (ticarcillin), 138
ticarcillin, 138
TICLID (ticlopidine), 80
ticlopidine, 80
tigecycline, 144
tiludronate, 226
timolol, 55, 67
tinzaparin, 81
tiotropium, 45, 210
tipranavir, 163
tizanidine, 52
TNKase (tenecteplase), 83
tobramycin, 143
tocainide, 74
tocilizumab, 221
TOFRANIL (imipramine), 101
tolazoline, 53
tolcapone, 111
TOLECTIN (tolmetin), 217
tolerance, 93
tolmetin, 217
tolterodine, 44
TONOCARD (tocainide), 74
topiramate, 116
TORISEL (temsirolimus), 180
TORADOL (ketorolac), 216
torcetrapib, 88
toremifene, 179, 189, 191
torsemide, 60
tositumomab, 178
TOVIAZ (fesoterodine), 44
toxicology, 228
TRACLEER (bosentan), 211
TRACRIUM (atracurium), 46
tramadol, 117
TRANDATE (labetalol), 55
trandolapril, 63
transposons, 133
TRANXENE (clorazepate), 94
tranylcypromine, 100–101
trastuzumab, 178
trazodone, 101, 104
TREANDA (bendamustine), 175
TRECATOR-SC (ethionamide), 151
treprostinil, 211
TRELSTAR (triptorelin), 179, 194
tretinoin, 181
trematodes, 159
TRENTAL (pentoxifylline), 84
TREXAN (naltrexone), 117
triamcinolone, 186, 209
triazolam, 94

TRILEPTAL (oxcarbazepine), 114
trimazosin, 53
trimethoprim, 134–135, 147
TRIMPEX (trimethoprim), 134–135, 147
triptorelin, 179, 194
troleandomycin, 145
tropicamide, 44
trospium, 44
tuberculosis, 151
tubocurarine, 46
tubular reabsorption, 25
tubular secretion, 25
tubulin, 160
TYGACIL (tigecycline), 144
TYKERB (lapatinib), 178
TYLENOL (acetaminophen), 220
TYSABRI (natalizumab), 215
TYZEKA (telbivudine), 165

ulcerative colitis, 214
ULORIC (febuxostat), 221
ULTRALENTE (insulin), 199
ULTRAM (tramadol), 117
URECHOLINE (bethanechol), 39
uric acid, 153
URISED (methenamine), 150
URO-PHOSPHATE (methenamine), 150
urokinase, 83
UROXATRAL (alfuzosin), 53

valacyclovir, 165
VALCYTE (valganciclovir), 165
valdecoxib, 218
valganciclovir, 165
VALIUM (diazepam), 64, 94
valsartan, 63
VALTREX (valacyclovir), 165
VANCOCIN (vancomycin), 134, 141
vancomycin, 134, 141
VASOTEC (enalapril), 63
VECTIBIX (panitumumab), 178
vecuronium, 46
VEETIDS (penicillin V), 138
VELBAN (vinblastine), 176
VELCADE (bortezomib), 180
VELSAR (vinblastine), 176
venlafaxine, 101–102

VENTAVIS (iloprost), 211
VENTOLIN (albuterol), 49, 209
VEPESIOL (etoposide), 176
verapamil, 64
VERMOX (mebendazole), 159
VERSED (midazolam), 125
VESANOID (tretinoin), 181
VESICARE (solifenacin), 44
VESTRA (reboxetine), 101
VFEND (voriconazole), 155
VIBATIV (telavancin), 141
VIBRAMYCIN (doxycycline), 144
VICTOZA (liraglutide), 201
vidarabine, 165
VIDEX (didanosine), 163
VIMPAT (lacosamide), 116
vinblastine, 176–177
vinorelbine, 176–177
VIOXX (rofecoxib), 218
VIRA-A (vidarabine), 165
VIRAMUNE (nevirapine), 163
VIRAZOLE (ribavirin), 165
VIREAD (tenofovir), 163
VISTARIL (hydroxyzine), 205
vitamin K, 82, 229–230
VOLTAREN (diclofenac), 216
voriconazole, 155
vorinostat, 181
VOTRIENT (pazopanib), 180
VUMOR (teniposide), 176

warfarin, 80–82
WELLBUTRIN (bupropion), 101
WELCHOL (colesevelam), 87, 201
whipworm, 160
WIGRAINE (ergotamine), 222
withdrawal, 93–94, 96–97
WYTENSIN (guanabenz), 52

XANAX (alprazolam), 94
XELODA (capecitabine), 176
XENICAL (orlistat), 215
XIGRIS (drotrecogin alfa), 81
ximelagatran, 84
XOLAIR (omalizumab), 210
XOPENEX (levalbuterol), 209
XYLOCAINE (lidocaine), 74–75, 77

XYROX (linezolid), 145
XYZAL (levocetirizine), 206

YOCON (yohimbine), 53
YODOXIN (iodoquinol), 167
yohimbine, 53

zaleplon, 94, 98
ZANAFLEX (tizanidine), 52
zanamivir, 164
ZANTAC (ranitidine), 213
ZARONTIN (ethosuximide),
    114–115
ZAROXOLYN (metolazone), 60
ZEBETA (bisoprolol), 55, 67
ZELDOX (ziprasidone), 107
ZEMPLAR (paricalcitol), 198
ZENAPAX (daclizumab),
    223–224
ZEVALIN (ibritumomab tiuxetan), 178
ZERIT (stavudine), 163
zero order, 115, 219
ZESTRIL (lisinopril), 63
ZETIA (ezetimibe), 87–88
ZIAGEN (abacavir), 163
zidovudine, 163
ZINECARD (dexrazoxane), 177
zileuton, 209
ziprasidone, 107
ZITHROMAX (azithromycin), 145
ZOCOR (simvastatin), 86
ZOLADEX (goserelin), 194
zoledronate, 226
ZOLINZA (vorinostat), 181
zolmitriptan, 222
ZOLOFT (sertraline), 101
zolpidem, 94, 98–99
ZOMETA (zoledronate), 226
ZOMIG (zolmitriptan), 222
ZONEGRAN (zonisamide), 116
zonisamide, 116
ZOVIRAX (acyclovir), 165
ZYBAN (bupropion), 101, 104
ZYFLO (zileuton), 209
ZYLOPRIM (allopurinol), 221–222
ZYPREXA (olanzapine), 107
ZYRTEC (cetirizine), 206–207